Laparoscopic Adjustable Gastric Banding

Laparoscopic Adjustable Gastric Banding

Achieving Permanent Weight Loss with Minimally Invasive Surgery

Jessie H. Ahroni, Ph.D., A.R.N.P.

iUniverse, Inc.

New York Lincoln Shanghai

Laparoscopic Adjustable Gastric Banding
Achieving Permanent Weight Loss with Minimally Invasive Surgery

iUniverse, Inc.

For information address:
iUniverse, Inc.
2021 Pine Lake Road, Suite 100
Lincoln, NE 68512
www.iuniverse.com

Cover image used with permission of the INAMED corporation.

ISBN: 0-595-31114-8 (pbk)
ISBN: 0-595-66262-5 (cloth)

Printed in the United States of America

CONTENTS

▼

Introduction... xi

Disclaimer xiii

Chapter 1:   The Obesity Epidemic... 1

What is Obesity? 1

What are the treatments for obesity?...2

    Dieting 2

    Exercise...2

    Over-the counter-medications 3

    Prescription medications..3

    Other methods..3

    Weight-loss surgery..4

Chapter 2:   Weight-loss Surgery 5

Main Types 5

    Gastric bypass...5

    Stomach stapling 7

    Adjustable gastric banding (AGB) 8

    Other surgeries...9

Why aren't more of these surgeries being performed? 10

Who is a candidate for surgery? 11

What are the specific criteria for weight-loss surgery?...........................12

How are these surgeries done? 13

Jessie's Story 14

Chapter 3:   Laparoscopic Adjustable Gastric Banding.......................17

Is laparoscopic adjustable gastric banding for you? 17

How does adjustable gastric banding work?...18

Is gastric banding painful? 18

What kind of scars will I have after gastric banding?....................................19

Where is the port placed? 19

Is gastric banding permanent? 20

How do I find a surgeon? 20

Do I need to see other health care professionals? 22

How does one decide if this is right for them? 22

Karen's Story..24

What are the contraindications for gastric banding? 25

What else can I do to find out more about weight-loss surgery?....................27

Chapter 4:   Benefits and Risks 29

What are the potential benefits of weight-loss surgery? 29

   Improved physical status..29

   Improved psychological status 29

   Relationships 30

   Self-esteem and body image 30

Becca's Story 30

How risky is gastric banding? 31

General surgical risks...31

Complications of gastric banding 32

Other complications..34

Chapter 5:   Dealing with Others..36

Should I tell my friends and family about this?...36

My family and friends are not supportive 37

How do I go about dealing with the health insurance company? 39

Toni's Story 39

Chapter 6:   Having Surgery and the First Few Weeks 41

Is there anything I should do before surgery? 41

How long do I have to stay in the hospital? 42

What tests are associated with gastric banding? 42

What is the immediate post-op recovery period like? 43

Why can't I smoke after surgery? 44

When can I return to work? 44

What can I have during the liquid phase of the post-op diet? 45

Clear Liquid Diet 47

Full Liquid Diet 48

Soft Diet 50

Why can't I have carbonated beverages after surgery? 52

What can I have during the soft foods phase of the post-op diet? 52

Chapter 7:   Adjusting the Adjustable Gastric Band 54

What is a band adjustment? 54

How is an adjustment done? 54

When do I have the first adjustment? 56

How many adjustments are needed? 56

How do I know if I need to have fluid let out? 57

How can I tell if I am perfectly adjusted? 57

Questions to determine if you need an eating adjustment 58

Questions to determine if you need a behavior adjustment 60

Questions to determine if you need an activity adjustment 61

Questions to determine if you need an attitude adjustment 62

Questions to determine if you need a band adjustment 63

Questions to determine if you need your band loosened 64

When to see your health care provider immediately 65

Chapter 8:   Eating after Gastric Banding 66

What can I eat? 66

How do I go about introducing solid foods back into my meals? 67

What foods should be avoided? 67

What else can I do to maximize my chances for weight loss success? 68

What should I be eating? 70

How long do I have to follow this diet? 72

What do you mean about changing your thinking? 72

How much can I eat? 73

Do I have to take vitamins? 74

What is dumping syndrome and do I have to worry about this? 74

Can I eat meat? 75

What's the problem with fiber? 75

Why can't I eat bread? 76

Should I be on a high-protein diet? 76

Should I be on a low-carbohydrate diet? 77

What is the glycemic index and does it matter? 77

Why can't I have high calorie liquids? 78

What is ketosis and how is it related to gastric banding? 78

Am I going to have trouble taking my medications? 79

Can I drink alcohol after surgery? 80

How often should I expect vomiting? 80

What if I have to vomit from having the flu or something? 81

Am I going to be constipated after surgery? 81

Chapter 9:   Follow-Up Care 83

What kind of medical follow-up will I need after gastric banding? 83

Will I have to exercise after surgery? 83

Patti's Story 84

What if I get pregnant? 87

Where can I find a support group for people with adjustable gastric bands?...........87

How much can I expect to lose? 88

Is adjustable gastric banding effective? 89

What weight loss can one expect with an adjustable gastric band? 90

Do people ever lose too much weight with gastric banding? 90

What is the "window of opportunity?" 91

Will I need a tummy tuck? 91

What happens to the band when I experience pressure changes?...........................92

Can you go scuba diving with a gastric band? 92

What happens if I become sick?...93

Getting on with the rest of your life..93

Bob's Story 93

Chapter 10:   More About Obesity..**96**

What are the causes of obesity? 96

Genetics and Heredity..*96*

Lifestyle...*97*

Psychology *97*

Overeating *98*

Metabolic disorders *98*

What is the "thrifty gene" theory and how is it related to obesity? 98

What are the risks of obesity?..99

Lung and breathing problems..*100*

Gallstones, heartburn, liver disease...*100*

Hypertension (high blood pressure)...*100*

Heart and coronary artery disease *100*

Strokes *101*

High cholesterol...*101*

Diabetes mellitus *101*

Arthritis, back and joint pain..*101*

Sexual and reproductive problems...*102*

Depression *102*

Cancer.. *102*

Mortality *102*

How serious a health problem is obesity?... 103

What other problems are associated with obesity? 103

What are the benefits of obesity? 106

Appendix 108

How do you figure your body mass index? 108

Body Mass Index Table... 109

BMI examples 111

Is the BMI calculation accurate? 112

Why does BMI matter? 113

What is ideal body weight? 113

Introduction

In modern society being and remaining slim or of normal weight receives much attention in the media for a variety of reasons. Millions of people throughout the world are attempting to reduce and control their weight, with varying degrees of success. Despite all the attention given to weight control, there has been a considerable increase in the number of people who are seriously overweight. Currently an estimated 67 percent of US adults are overweight or obese, along with 13 percent of children and adolescents. The prevalence of serious obesity among US adults is about 20 percent, which reflects a 61 percent increase since 1991.

Being seriously overweight or severely obese can cause physical problems and diseases, such as heart disease and diabetes. It may also have major psychological consequences such as a negative self-image and social isolation.

No doubt you already know the best remedy for excess weight: eat less and exercise more. Essentially this means eating small portions and choosing lower calorie foods more frequently. You may have tried to burn more calories by increasing your activity level dramatically. You have probably tried eating less and exercising more several times. Sometimes you may have even been very successful. But you found that although these methods do indeed show results in the short term, as soon as you stop the program you go back up to your old weight or even end up weighing more than you did prior to your weight-loss attempts.

Drugs that suppress your appetite do not usually result in lasting weight loss. If you have already tried everything and found that none of these methods helped you to permanently lose your excess weight, you may be ready for weight-loss surgery. Surgery to reduce the amount of food you can eat may be your only remaining option. These pages tell you about the surgical options for losing weight. Although other surgeries are discussed a bit, the primary focus of this book is laparoscopic adjustable gastric banding.

Disclaimer

The purpose of this book is to acquaint you with weight-loss surgery and with laparoscopic adjustable gastric banding. The information, services, products, messages, and other materials contained here are provided for educational and general information purposes only and are not a substitute for medical advice and treatment. The inclusion of medical information is not intended to create a caregiver-patient relationship. The answers are for informational purposes only. They do not imply diagnosis or treatment and should always be used in conjunction with the advice of your personal health care provider. Any representation contained here is not intended to expressly or impliedly warrant or create any standard of care. Once again, it is not intended to replace medical advice from your health care provider.

CHAPTER 1

▼

THE OBESITY EPIDEMIC

WHAT IS OBESITY?

Being overweight is defined as weighing 10 or 20 pounds more than the recommended weight for your height. Obesity is often defined as being 20 or 30% or more over ideal body weight. Obesity affects an estimated 34 million Americans. It is very common. In some circles it is being called an epidemic.

Morbid obesity is a more severe form of obesity in which a person is 100 or more pounds overweight. Morbid obesity affects an estimated four million Americans. Sometimes morbid obesity is defined as being more than 150% of your ideal body weight. Morbid obesity affects every area of a person's life.

Obesity is not a behavioral problem or character flaw. Obesity is recognized by the National Institutes of Health as a disease. Obesity has profoundly negative health and social consequences. The medical problems caused or made worse by obesity are numerous, serious, and often life-threatening.

WHAT ARE THE TREATMENTS FOR OBESITY?

Dieting

Because of the negative health and social implications of obesity, people often seek treatment. The most common form of treatment is dieting. Dieting, however, is rarely successful in the long term, especially if a person is morbidly obese. The success rate for dieting is approximately 3 to 5 percent. In other words, 95 to 97% of people who try dieting fail to lose weight permanently.

I'm not saying diets don't work. They do work, but only for as long as you stay on them. Once you quit dieting and go back to eating in the usual way most people regain all the weight they lost and then some.

When this cycle is repeated frequently it is called the "yo-yo" effect. Dieting, regaining weight, dieting again, regaining again, can make it harder to lose weight in the future. This type of cyclical dieting mimics the effects of repeated famines. The body becomes more efficient at using and storing calories and protects itself against weight loss as a result of yo-yo dieting.

Exercise

As a weight loss strategy, exercise is not as potent as dieting. A look at any table of how many calories are burned with certain types of exercise will tell you that you have to do an awful lot of exercise to significantly affect your weight. Exercise combined with dieting leads to more weight loss than using either strategy alone. However, exercise isn't very effective, and it is effective only as long as you do it. Once you go back to your ordinary lifestyle the weight you lost while exercising is usually regained.

This does not mean exercise is bad or worthless. Exercising and being physically fit are definitely good for you. Exercise is more effective in reshaping your body than it is for losing excess weight. Exercise can help build muscles, and muscles burn calories for fuel. However, exercise isn't a permanent solution to obesity.

Over-the counter-medications

There are many items in drugstores and health food stores that claim to help people lose weight. None seem to be both safe and effective. The ones that are effective are only minimally so, and they have significant side effects and health risks. The ones that are safe do not seem to be very effective in helping folks lose weight and keep it off. Think about it: if there really were a safe and effective weight loss product available over the counter, almost everyone would be thin.

Prescription medications

In spite of a tremendous amount of research, there still is no magic pill that melts pounds away effortlessly. Obese people and their health care providers had great hopes for fen-phen (fenfluramine and phentermine) a combination stimulant and antidepressant, but those hopes were dashed when some of the people taking it developed heart problems. New medications are available, and more are in the pipeline. Talk to your doctor about their pros and cons.

Even if an effective weight loss drug were found tomorrow, would you really want to take medication for the rest of your life to maintain your weight? Because obesity is such a complex problem, a prescription medication may work for some, but not for others. Your body has many complex mechanisms and backup systems to maintain weight. A drug that would affect all of these without significant side effects seems unlikely. Do you have 10 years to wait for an effective drug to be developed, tested and proven safe?

Other methods

Other options such as counseling, jaw wiring, and hypnosis may help with weight loss in the short term, but when used alone these methods are rarely effective for permanent weight loss.

Weight-loss surgery

Currently, the most effective form of therapy for morbid obesity is surgery. It is true that diet, exercise and medications can help, but they will not usually help a person lose as much weight, nor will the weight loss be as long-term as with surgery.

Not everyone who has a weight problem should consider surgery. Surgery is not an easy way to help you lose a few pounds. It is a serious treatment for a serious disease, not a cosmetic procedure.

Even surgery is not a guarantee. Surgery can help you achieve long-term weight loss only if you are ready for and committed to losing weight and keeping it off. Even if you have surgery you will still have to eat less and be more physically active. Surgery alone is not effective, and it is possible to have surgery and still not lose much weight if you do not also make the necessary lifestyle changes. You will have to adapt to a different way of life.

CHAPTER 2

▼

WEIGHT-LOSS SURGERY

WHAT ARE THE MAIN TYPES OF WEIGHT-LOSS SURGERY?

There are several different types of weight-loss surgery that aim to accomplish one or both of two basic purposes: (1) limiting the amount of food you can eat and (2) limiting the amount of nutrients your body can absorb. The American Society for Bariatric Surgery recently estimated that 63,100 Americans per year chose surgical methods such as stomach stapling, gastric bypass surgery and gastric banding to permanently reduce their weight.

These surgeries are generally considered a last resort as a treatment for obesity and are usually done only after other programs have been seriously tried and found to be unsuccessful. Your doctor or insurance company may want you to document the other types of weight loss programs you have tried or to seriously try diet and exercise one more time before considering surgery.

Gastric bypass

Gastric bypass is both a restrictive and a malabsorptive procedure. Common types of gastric bypasses are the Roux-en-Y (RNY), the Billroth II loop bypass and the duodenal switch (DS). These surgeries are similar but there are important differences as to just what is bypassed and where the connections are made. If you are considering one of these surgeries, you will need to have a surgeon explain exactly what is to be done. Each surgeon may take a slightly different approach. Below is a general description.

A gastric bypass is essentially what it sounds like. A very small stomach pouch is created. The major portion of the stomach and some of the intestines are bypassed. A short segment of intestine is connected directly to the small stomach pouch. Because of the small stomach pouch, a person with a gastric bypass can eat only small amounts. Because the intestines are bypassed some of what is eaten is not digested or absorbed.

Generally people with a gastric bypass tolerate sweets poorly. If they eat things with a significant amount of concentrated sugar or fat, they may experience a syndrome called "dumping" when these substances contact the intestines. Common symptoms include feeling lightheaded, having palpitations or a rapid pulse, and sweating. These symptoms usually only last a short while, but they are very unpleasant, so people with this surgery become conditioned against eating sweets and concentrated fat. However not all gastric bypass patients experience dumping syndrome and you should not go into this surgery counting on dumping syndrome to keep you from eating the wrong thing. Even if you have dumping syndrome at first, your body may be able to tolerate these substances over time and the effects of dumping may wear off.

Because a gastric bypass causes malabsorption, the potential for long-term complications is greater than with other surgeries. After a bypass an individual can experience low protein levels, anemia, vitamin deficiencies, or low calcium levels. Many bypass surgery patients have to take protein, vitamin, or mineral supplements every day for the rest of their lives to avoid these problems. There are many variations on the gastric bypass surgery, but essentially they all perform in a similar fashion.

Most modern gastric bypass surgeries are technically reversible, although this depends to some degree on exactly what was done. Generally the stitches or staples that made the stomach smaller can be removed and the stomach and intestines can be reconnected similar to the way they were before surgery. Generally all the weight lost will be regained if the gastric bypass is reversed.

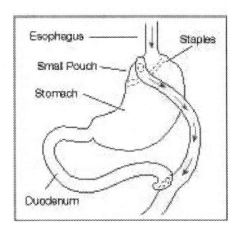

Stomach stapling

This procedure is a restrictive surgery. A small stomach pouch is created at the top of the stomach by partitioning the stomach with sutures (stitches) or staples. The outlet from this pouch is carefully measured and a small band is placed around the outlet.

This procedure is called a vertical banded gastroplasty (VBG). Gastro means stomach. Plasty means changing the shape of. Vertical refers to the fact the staples are placed up and down. Banded refers to the band around the pouch outlet. Vertical banded gastroplasty is abbreviated VBG.

This operation causes weight loss by forcing the patients to eat small meals. If these patients overeat, they will vomit.

A major disadvantage of the VBG is that fluids pass through the pouch easily. If the patient consumes high-calorie fluids such as milk shakes and fruit juice, not much weight will be lost. Over time, the pouch may stretch or the staple line may break down.

This surgery is also technically reversible. The stitches or staples and the band placed around the outlet can usually be removed. Generally all the weight lost will be regained if the VBG is reversed.

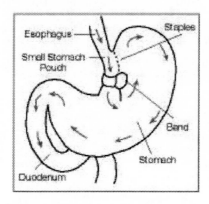

Adjustable gastric banding (AGB)

Adjustable gastric banding involves applying a band around the upper part of the stomach. This creates a small gastric pouch at the top of the stomach with a small opening to the rest of the stomach. The band is made of an inflatable ring that controls the flow of food from the small pouch to the rest of the digestive tract. In other words the stomach will be hourglass shaped after the surgery. There is no cutting or stapling needed to divide the stomach.

A small port is connected by a length of tubing to the inflatable ring around the stomach. The port is placed just beneath the skin where fluid can be injected or withdrawn to adjust the size of the opening between the upper and lower portions of the stomach. Adjustable gastric banding is abbreviated AGB.

Like the stomach stapling, a major disadvantage of banding is that fluids pass through the pouch easily. If the patient consumes high calorie fluids such as milk shakes and fruit juice then not much weight will be lost. Unlike the stomach stapling, the gastric band can be adjusted to accommodate each patient's individual situation. Generally the band is made tighter with time. As you lose weight you also lose fat around the stomach, the stomach shrinks, the pouch can stretch a bit, and some people think the stomach wall becomes thinner. Adding fluid to the band will decrease the size of the opening between the upper and lower portions of the stomach.

If for some reason one needed to eat more, the effects of the band can be greatly reduced by just withdrawing the fluid from the balloon with a needle through the skin. Loosening the band opens up the portal between the upper and lower stomach. The band can also be removed if necessary. Generally all the weight lost will be regained if the band is removed.

In the United States, the FDA approved adjustable gastric banding surgery in June of 2001. However, the band is not a new invention. It was developed in the 1980s and has been used in Europe since 1993. There are a growing number of places in the US where experienced surgeons are placing gastric bands. Many North Americans who wanted a gastric band before it was FDA-approved went outside the USA for the surgery. The surgery is readily available in Europe, Mexico, Latin America, the Mideast, and Australia.

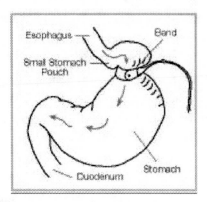

Other surgeries

Although these are the three main types of weight-loss surgery currently available, there are other variations that are beyond the scope of this book. The focus of this book is the adjustable gastric banding surgery and comments from this point forward will be specifically directed toward that procedure only.

IF THE DATA ABOUT WEIGHT-LOSS SURGERY ARE SO CONVINCING WHY AREN'T MORE OF THESE SURGERIES BEING PERFORMED?

There are several reasons why weight-loss surgery has not been very popular. There are few surgeons who are trained to treat obesity and even fewer who are trained in the after care of an obesity surgery patient. For most types of surgery, the surgeons perform an operation on a patient and after the patient heals from the surgery they will not see the surgeons again unless they need a second procedure. Most surgeons' practices are not set up to provide the long term follow-up, patient education, and behavior change support the way medical practices for chronic diseases like diabetes might be.

Society discriminates against people with obesity because there is a failure to understand that obesity needs ongoing treatment just like any other disease. There is also prejudice against surgeons who carry out this type of surgery. Some doctors consider surgery for obesity to be a waste of resources and others remember the poor results from earlier weight loss surgeries that had high rates of complications, failure, and death.

Many people who have had weight-loss surgery are reluctant to talk about their procedure with others who may not have known them when they were obese. They do not advertise the benefits the way people who are cured from other terminal diseases might. There is a lack of robust data on the costs and benefits of weight-loss surgery, although it has been suggested that even modest weight loss will decrease co-morbidities (other medical problems that are being caused or made worse by obesity). The benefits of weight-loss surgery have not been researched and documented in medical literature as well as they should be. This is gradually changing, but until high-quality studies are published in mainstream medical literature, many physicians do not believe or know about the effectiveness of weight-loss surgery. Many medical doctors don't know much about weight-loss surgery and have few patients who have experienced the benefits. In the United States there is a prejudice in the medical community against accepting research from other countries as being reliable.

Some health care insurance providers will not pay for weight-loss surgery because they do not understand or believe that the procedures are cost effective in the long run. Many insurance companies exclude all treatments for obesity from coverage.

For these reasons weight-loss surgery has been driven into the private sector where only the rich can benefit. It is expected that this will change in the coming years. More surgeons will be trained to perform these life saving operations, medical care will be restructured to provide the follow-up that is required to help patients make and sustain the behavior change that accompanies profound weight loss, and insurance coverage will become available. Several excellent research studies of weight-loss surgery are now underway and will soon be published. Once treatment for obesity is accepted like treatment for any other disease, people will be more willing to talk about it and—hopefully—some of the prejudice will end.

WHO IS A CANDIDATE FOR SURGERY?

In general, weight-loss surgeries are designed for severely obese people who are between 16 and 60 years old and who have attempted dieting, exercise programs and medical management of their obesity but have been unsuccessful in maintaining permanent weight loss. Many candidates for surgery have co-morbidities that are being caused or made worse by obesity.

These age limits are somewhat arbitrary. It is not usually considered a good idea to perform weight-loss surgery until someone has finished growing and until they are mature enough to deal with the restrictions imposed by surgery, establish a sensible eating plan and maintain it for the rest of their life.

Older people can have weight-loss surgery. Many times people over 60 will have other health problems that make the surgery riskier. Some of the benefits of weight-loss surgery such as preventing heart disease, diabetes, and other complications of obesity are less effective in older people because they may already have these complications established, especially if they have been obese for many years. Some older people may find it harder to

change life-long habits, thus undermining the surgery. You must be willing to change your thinking and your habits to make weight-loss surgery
work for you. The benefits of being more active may not be as great for
older people because it is unlikely and may even be dangerous for them to
become extremely active, especially if they have never been active before.

If you do not fall within the age requirements but you think you might
benefit from weight-loss surgery you should discuss your situation with
your doctors.

WHAT ARE THE SPECIFIC CRITERIA FOR WEIGHT-LOSS SURGERY?

Each surgeon or surgical center will have specific criteria for weight-loss
surgery. Your surgeon's requirements may be different than what is stated
here. Most surgeons follow the recommendations from the 1991 National
Institutes of Health Consensus Development Conference Statement on
the surgical treatment of obesity.

In general, to qualify for weight-loss surgery you must be at least 100
pounds overweight, 150% of ideal body weight or have a body mass index
greater than 40. You can find a chart in the appendix that can help you figure your body mass index (BMI).

In certain circumstances, less severely obese patients (with BMI's
between 35 and 40) also may be considered for surgery. Included in this
category are patients with high-risk co-morbid conditions such as
life-threatening severe sleep apnea, obesity-related heart problems, or
severe diabetes mellitus. Other possible indications for patients with BMI's
between 35 and 40 include obesity-induced physical problems that are
interfering with lifestyle (e.g. musculo-skeletal, neurological, or body size
problems precluding or severely interfering with employment, family
function and ambulation).

The specific criteria are:

- You have been overweight for five years or more.

- You have made serious attempts to lose weight in the past and have had only short-term success. It is up to your doctor and your insurance company to define what constitutes a "serious" attempt. Generally a doctor-supervised program that you followed for a year would be considered a serious attempt. Joining a gym for a few weeks would probably be considered a less serious attempt.

- You do not have any other disease that may have caused you to be overweight (like hypothyroidism), or if you do it is under treatment.

- You are willing, able, and prepared to make major changes in your eating habits and lifestyle. A person who states they are willing to make healthy food choices and to deal with their emotions directly rather than resort to emotional eating would be considered a better candidate than someone who states they do not wish to give up eating at fast food restaurants.

- You are willing to work with the specialists who are treating you during the post-surgical period to get proper follow-up care.

- You do not drink alcohol or use drugs to excess.

- If you don't meet these criteria but still feel you might benefit from weight-loss surgery, go ahead and contact a surgeon. There are exceptions.

HOW ARE THESE SURGERIES DONE?

Generally all of the weight loss surgeries can either be performed laparoscopically or in a traditional open procedure with an incision in the abdomen. Not all surgeons are trained in laparoscopic surgery. Laparoscopic surgery is also known as keyhole surgery. It involves inserting several trocars into the abdomen after the abdomen has been inflated with carbon dioxide gas. Trocars are hollow tubes. The surgery is then performed with special thin instruments and a thin camera through the trocars. The pictures from the camera are watched on a TV screen. Laparoscopic surgery is usually considered more technically difficult to perform and may be more expensive than open surgery. This type of laparoscopic surgery requires general anesthesia.

Laparoscopic surgery leaves smaller scars and the recovery time is generally faster than after traditional surgery. Patients normally leave the hospital one to three days after surgery.

Whether or not you will be able to have laparoscopic surgery depends on several things. Generally the heavier you are and the more complex your procedure the less likely you are to have laparoscopic surgery. Even if you go into surgery believing that you are having a laparoscopic procedure there may be technical difficulties during the procedure that make it necessary for the surgeon to convert to an open abdominal incision. The anatomy of each individual varies greatly. You and your surgeon will need to discuss this thoroughly before the operation so that you understand both the plan and what might happen if the plan does not work out.

JESSIE'S STORY

Although this whole book is everything I've learned about adjustable gastric banding since I first heard of the procedure, this is my weight-loss story.

I never in my wildest dreams ever thought that I would weigh over 200 pounds. And then I weighed 205, then 210 and 215, and then I stopped weighing. I knew something had to change. Being a research nurse practitioner had taught me to search the medical literature so I began a quest to find out what treatments were actually effective for permanent weight loss. I'd already lost many pounds many times on various diets and programs and even kept the weight off for years at a time occasionally. But the weight always came back, bringing 10 or 15 friends (more pounds) with it. At this point my blood sugar was creeping up. My father had diabetes, and I was a diabetes educator and worked in diabetes research. I knew this was one disease I didn't want. I also knew the only way to prevent diabetes was to lose weight. However, that wasn't my main goal. I was tired of being single. And I knew I'd have a lot more dating options at my age if I weighed less.

It didn't take me long to come to the conclusion that weight-loss surgery was the only effective treatment for obesity. Once I realized that, I began to research surgical options and soon discovered gastric banding. It immediately looked like a simple and elegant solution to me that might actually work. I spent the next few weeks spending every spare minute reading everything I could find about adjustable gastric banding, both in the medical and the lay literature and on the Internet.

On October 3, 1998, a few weeks before my 50th birthday, I was banded. Over the next 9 months I lost 85 pounds, bringing my weight from 218 to 133 pounds. I still haven't developed diabetes (although my younger sister who is still obese has) and in August of 2001 I married my new husband. So yes, you can say I met my weight loss goals, but there was so much more to the journey than just being healthier, thinner and having a mate.

At first I didn't tell anybody that I had weight-loss surgery. The one friend I confided in was very negative about the whole idea and didn't really understand the difference between gastric banding and other more radical procedures. I worked in a huge medical clinic with a lot of people who had a tendency toward gossip and I just didn't want people watching me and talking about me. After I had lost 30 or 40 pounds people would ask, "How are you losing so much weight?" I would say, "Well, I eat less and I exercise more" (which was basically the truth). After I'd been successful for a year and was pretty sure the weight was going to stay off, I did confess that I'd had weight-loss surgery.

Getting the weight out of the way freed me to deal with other important issues in my life. I learned to quit spending my time and thoughts obsessing about my weight and what I was eating or wasn't eating or shouldn't eat or wished I could eat. I stopped getting on the scale every morning and letting the scale determine if I was having a good day or a bad day. I gradually learned to work with the band to control my intake. I learned to be satisfied with eating less and to find other pleasures in my life. I also had to learn that rather than eat when I was tired, bored, lonely, frustrated, anxious, angry, sad or happy that there were other more appropriate ways to deal with those emotions.

This wasn't easy. Back in the days when I was banded I only knew two other women who had this surgery. We formed our own little support group and—through the Internet—invited others to join us. We also participated in online support groups. When I had problems or met obstacles, I would discuss it with my support group friends. With their love and assistance I learned to figure out what I really wanted out of life and decided what I was willing to do to get it. I've been able to keep my weight within the normal range for more than five years. When my research grants suddenly ended due to cutbacks in federal funding—and I found myself needing a new job—it seemed like a natural extension of my passion to join a weight-loss surgery practice. And now it's a daily pleasure to help other people successfully lose weight with gastric banding.

▼

Laparoscopic Adjustable Gastric Banding

Is laparoscopic adjustable gastric banding for you?

For people who have tried everything and remain severely obese, or for people who have an obesity-related disease, surgery may be the best option. For other people, who are not severely obese, greater efforts towards weight control, such as changes in eating habits, and increasing physical activity may deserve another try. Ask yourself these questions:

- How many serious weight loss attempts have you tried?

- Are you unlikely to lose weight successfully with diet and exercise?

- Do you have a BMI of 40 or more?

- Do you have obesity-related physical problems or high-risk obesity-related health problems?

- Are you aware of how your life might change after the operation?

- Are you willing and able to make the necessary adjustments in your thinking, eating behaviors, activity levels and lifestyle?

- Are you aware of the potential for serious complications, the associated dietary restrictions and the possibility of failure?

- Are you committed to losing weight permanently?

HOW DOES ADJUSTABLE GASTRIC BANDING WORK?

The gastric band limits how much you can eat, reduces your appetite and slows digestion. This alone will not solve your weight problem but it can be a big help. Remember, gastric banding does not guarantee that you will lose weight. You will have to change your eating habits to lose weight with this device.

IS GASTRIC BANDING PAINFUL?

The amount of pain you experience after surgery varies greatly from person to person. Generally you will feel a bit of pain or discomfort. For most people ordinary painkillers will provide relief during the first few days to a week. People rarely need pain medication longer than a few days after laparoscopic surgery. If you had to have open surgery or other procedures performed at the same time you may have more pain.

Most people who have a gastric band placed laparoscopically are able to get out of bed and walk around a few hours after surgery. This helps prevent blood clots, respiratory problems and bedsores. Even if you had your gall bladder removed or a hernia repaired at the same time you'll probably be getting out of bed the same day you had surgery.

During laparoscopic surgery the abdomen is filled with carbon dioxide gas to lift up the skin, separate the organs and make more room for the surgeon to work. They will try to remove most of this gas before closing your surgical wounds but a small amount may remain. Your body will reabsorb any remaining gas quickly. Inflating the abdomen in this way tends to stretch the diaphragm. This creates a special type of pain called "referred pain" which is felt in the left shoulder. Even though the problem is the stretched muscle of the diaphragm the pain is felt in the shoulder because of the way the nerves in this area are connected. It does not mean anything is wrong with your shoulder. This pain varies from little or none to more intense discomfort, but usually it can be controlled with pain medication. It will gradually go away after a few days. Heat to either the shoulder or the upper abdomen can be used to help relieve it. A shoulder massage may also provide relief.

WHAT KIND OF SCARS WILL I HAVE AFTER GASTRIC BANDING?

Yes, you will have scars after surgery. These can range from very small one-inch scars after a laparoscopic procedure to a much larger midline abdominal scar after an open procedure.

Generally people who have a laparoscopic adjustable gastric band end up with about 4 or 5 of these tiny scars plus a slightly larger one for the port placement. These tiny scars tend to heal well and after a few months or a year will be barely visible.

If you are concerned about this you can ask your surgeon about what kind of scar to expect. You might also find people at a support group meeting that would be willing to show you their scars so you will know what they look like.

WHERE IS THE PORT PLACED?

There are several common locations for port placement. One of the most common locations for a gastric band port is on the left side of the abdomen, below the ribcage and either above or below the waist. Another site that might be used is on the bottom of the sternum (breastbone) in the center of the chest. Each surgeon will have a plan for where he or she plans to place the port. You should discuss this with your surgeon before the operation. Sometimes the surgeon will want to mark where your belt or skirt goes around your waist or mark the bra line so that the port does not end up uncomfortably positioned under your garments. The port will be sutured in place to the muscle. As you lose weight the port may move a bit and tend to come to the surface as the overlying fat disappears. You will probably be able to feel it when you press on the spot but it shouldn't be painful or protuberant.

Some people have special reasons for having their port located in a different place and if you feel either of these sites would be a problem for you then you'll need to talk to your surgeon.

If the port ends up in a place that is difficult for you or difficult to access it can be moved. Sometimes moving the port can be done in the office or clinic under local anesthesia.

IS GASTRIC BANDING PERMANENT?

At the present time the gastric band is intended to be in place permanently. There are no known reasons to suggest it needs to be removed or replaced if no complications occur. If it is removed it is quite likely you will regain any weight that was lost. However since this device is relatively new to the market there is no guarantee that it will not have to be removed or replaced at some time in the future.

If the band has to be removed or replaced, generally this can be done laparoscopically. In most cases the stomach will probably return to an essentially normal shape after the band is removed.

HOW DO I FIND A SURGEON?

The doctors who perform weight-loss surgery are called bariatric surgeons or general surgeons. The best way to find one is to get a recommendation from someone else that has had successful weight-loss surgery. The next best place is to get a recommendation from your regular medical doctor.

You might want to check and see if your surgeon has completed a residency in this or a related specialty.

If you wish to have a laparoscopic adjustable gastric banding you will need to find a surgeon who is trained in laparoscopic surgery and has all the necessary equipment. Currently the manufacturer of the product must train surgeons who install the gastric band. The manufacturer maintains a list of surgeons authorized to use their device and you may be able to get the name of a local surgeon who has been trained in laparoscopic adjustable gastric banding from them.

I would not suggest that you pick a surgeon based solely on a listing in the Yellow Pages, advertising or mention by the media. Reputable surgeons do have to advertise for patients these days, but you should check out their credentials and not base your decision on only what you see in the ad.

In some states you can contact the state medical board and check to see if a doctor has any complaints or sanctions against him or her. Unless there are numerous complaints, this does not necessarily mean he or she is a bad surgeon, but it is just another factor you might what to check. Many surgeons will have complaints against them at some time in their careers, not necessarily because they did anything wrong. Sometimes patients have a bad outcome or are unhappy and will file a complaint.

Picking a surgeon is a very personal decision. It is important that you trust your surgeon's skills, support staff and bedside manner. Choose someone who you trust to give you good medical care, but also consider that this person can be a powerful ally in your weight loss journey. You should carefully assess how easy it is to talk to the surgeon and if you will feel comfortable discussing your weight loss struggles with this person over the long term.

Do not choose your surgeon by price alone.

Do I need to see other health care professionals?

Many surgeons who perform weight-loss surgery will have a team of professionals that they use to help patients. There will be a team of professionals in the operating room, recovery room and hospital or surgery center. These will include the surgeon, an assistant, an anesthesiologist and nurses and other health care professionals. Facilities that perform weight-loss surgery may or may not be set up to deal with obese patients. Those that are will have wide wheel chairs, large hospital gowns, and special tables and equipment. If you are worried about this you should ask your doctor what kinds of special equipment might be available at the hospital or surgical center.

There also will be a weight-loss surgery team that you will see before and after you leave the hospital. This team might include a nurse, dietician, exercise physiologist and a psychologist or weight-loss counselor. Your doctor may have several patients who form a support group to help each other before and after surgery. Ask about these resources early in your conversations with the surgeon. It is a good idea to attend a support group of patients who already have had the surgery before you have it so you can get all your questions answered from their perspective. Most surgeons will encourage you to do this.

If your surgeon does not employ the team approach you can seek out these kinds of help on your own if you have trouble with making a meal or activity plan or dealing with relationships or feelings about changing your body shape. Ask your doctor or other weight-loss surgery patients for a referral.

How does one decide if this is right for them?

Only you can decide if you want to pursue laparoscopic adjustable gastric banding as a method of permanent weight loss. The final decision will be made between you and your surgeon. However you should be aware that adjustable gastric banding is not an easy option or a quick fix to help you lose a few pounds. It is intended as a treatment for the serious disease of obesity. The success of band surgery depends on your ability to establish a sensible eating plan and maintain it for the rest of your life.

You need to have realistic expectations about any weight-loss surgery and how it works. Any unresolved issues relating to food or eating will still exist after surgery. If you think you have serious psychological issues that interfere with your ability to maintain new eating habits after surgery you should investigate these before deciding to have surgery.

You must realize that weight-loss surgery is not a guarantee of weight loss. It is possible to sabotage any surgery. Although weight-loss surgery will reduce hunger and the amount of solid food that can be consumed at one sitting, it is not a magic wand. The surgery is just one part of an over-all plan. Having weight-loss surgery is a permanent commitment to a change in lifestyle. If you are not ready or willing to change your lifestyle permanently, you should not have surgery.

It is also possible that you may not lose all of your excess weight. Talk to your surgeon about how much weight you can expect to lose. Generally speaking, most people lose between one-half and three-fourths of their excess weight, although some people lose 100%. Calculate what that means for you. For example if you are a 300-pound person who should weigh 150 pounds and you lose one third of your excess weight you would still weigh 250 pounds. If this theoretical person lost two-thirds of their excess weight, he or she would still weigh 200 pounds. You need to ask yourself if you would be satisfied with that degree of success after surgery. Even if you do not reach your desired weight the chances are good that your health and self-image will improve with significant surgical weight loss. You should spend some time before surgery deciding what a realistic weight is for you personally, rather than just relying on published tables.

KAREN'S STORY

All of my life I have struggled with my weight. I remember as a teen keeping a diary only allowing myself 500 calories a day in order to stay at a size 9 (I am 5'5"). During my 20's I was able to stay a size 14, however after the birth of my second child and the death of my husband (which happened within three months of each other) the pounds started to pile on. I don't remember going over 200 pounds, my memory only seems to remember being over 200 pounds. I was on a constant diet. You name it, I tried it. The only exercise I got consisted of walking around the neighborhood. In February 2001, I had a pulmonary embolism (blood clot in the lungs). I was one of the lucky ones, as 90% of pulmonary embolisms are diagnosed at autopsy. Ultrasounds, cat scans and MRI's could not find a blood clot in the leg, which is where most blood clots originate. I had no blood factor disorders. After seeing two specialists, the only advice I was given was to lose weight! Oh, how I wanted to. At that point I was 235 pounds, about a size 20. I looked into weight-loss surgery; however, I was not ready mentally to have an extreme surgical procedure done. Over the next few years I tried and tried to lose weight. I would be successful and would lose about 10 to 15 lbs, only to gain them back plus one or two more. I never really saw myself as fat, until I saw a picture of me in the summer of 2002! Oh my gosh! I was shocked! I really started walking at night and trying to watch what I ate. However, I had gained another 10 pounds! In March of 2003 I took a trip to Hawaii, the pictures revealed how much weight I really had on me. I couldn't believe how round I was. I didn't feel that fat, but the pictures didn't lie. Over the next few months I lost five pounds, gained five, lost five, and gained five. I was heading nowhere quickly. At a meeting in June I ran into a friend who had lost about 60 pounds. I hadn't seen her since November and she looked awesome! She confided in me that she had had a gastric bypass and gave me her doctor's name and phone number. I went home with some hope! I started researching weight-loss surgery again, but this time I was ready mentally. While searching the Internet, I ran into a personal website made by a lady who was banded. The light turned on and I started a detailed research project into the adjustable gastric band. After many months of research and talking to others who were banded, I had my surgery preformed on October 25, 2003 at the weight of 252 pounds. To date (five months), I have lost 60 pounds. This loss has not been without hard work on my emotional eating issues. I didn't realize how much I was really eating and for what reasons. Having the band placed has brought all of these issues to the forefront and has made me work on them. Not only has the band helped me change the way I view food and my relationship with it, it has helped me learn to love myself and who I am. My self-esteem is so much higher now. I am more outgoing. I have more energy now than time (it used to be I had more time than energy). I feel healthy and have no more daily aches and pains. I have 40 more pounds to lose to hit my goal; however I feel that I am a winner no matter where I end up on the scale because of the healthier me.

WHAT ARE THE CONTRAINDICATIONS FOR GASTRIC BANDING?

In addition to the general contraindications stated here, each surgeon or surgical center may have specific contraindications for weight-loss surgery. Your surgeon's rules may be different than what is stated here. If you have any of these problems, but you still think you might benefit from weight-loss surgery, you should discuss it with your health care providers.

Gastric banding may not be right for you if you have an inflammatory disease or condition of the gastrointestinal tract such as ulcers, esophagitis, or Crohn's disease.

Severe heart, lung or other disease that makes you a poor candidate for surgery would also be a contraindication.

If you have a problem that could cause excessive bleeding of the esophagus, stomach or intestines weight-loss surgery would not be recommended. This includes esophageal or gastric varices (dilated veins) and congenital or acquired intestinal telangiectasia (dilation of small blood vessels).

If your esophagus, stomach or intestines were not shaped normally (for example if you have narrowing of these) weight-loss surgery would be contraindicated.

A large unrepaired hiatal hernia could be a problem. This is when the top of the stomach protrudes up through the diaphragm muscle. The surgeon would not be able to place the gastric band in the right place in this instance. Sometimes a hiatal hernia can be repaired either before or during weight-loss surgery.

A gastric band is not placed while a person is pregnant. If you become pregnant after banding surgery the band may need to be deflated or in very rare cases even removed. The same is true if you need more nutrition for any other reason, such as becoming seriously ill. For example if you had cancer and chemotherapy and needed more nutrition, the band could be deflated until you recovered.

People who are addicted to drugs or alcohol are not good candidates for adjustable gastric banding.

If you have an infection that could contaminate the surgical area, you would not be a good candidate for surgery until the infection was completely resolved.

If you need to take aspirin or non-steroidal anti-inflammatory drugs, often this could conflict with gastric banding because these medications are stomach irritants. You might be able to switch to other drugs or other forms of these drugs that do not irritate the stomach, but you would need to discuss this fully with your health care providers before adjustable gastric banding would be considered.

If you cannot or do not want to follow the dietary restrictions that come with this surgery, then gastric banding is unlikely to work and you should not have the surgery. Generally, after gastric banding you will only be able to eat small amounts of food. You will have to chew your food well and stop eating at the very first hint that the small upper pouch might be full. There may be some foods that you cannot eat such as bread, tough meat, and fibrous vegetables. You should not drink with your meals and you cannot consume large quantities of soft or liquid calories, as they will run right through the band. Eating after gastric banding is discussed in greater detail later.

If you are allergic to materials in the device, that would be a contraindication.

Generally, the gastric band is painless once it is properly placed, but if you cannot tolerate any pain or discomfort from an implanted device, then the adjustable gastric band is not a good idea for you.

People who are not emotionally stable are not good candidates for any form of weight-loss surgery.

Adjustable gastric banding is not recommended for people who have an autoimmune connective tissue disease such as systemic lupus erythematosus or scleroderma.

Some surgeons believe that patients who are sweet eaters do not do well with the gastric banding. There is some research to support this idea, but there is also research that refutes it. Some surgeons might not do the surgery if you eat a lot of sweets and drink milk shakes and high-calorie liquids often. Other surgeons do not see this as a problem and look to the overall volume that you eat and whether or not you are willing to give up drinking high-calorie liquids.

WHAT ELSE CAN I DO TO FIND OUT MORE ABOUT WEIGHT-LOSS SURGERY?

In addition to reading this book, you need to interview some surgeons, go to any available support groups and ask to talk to patients who have had the surgery. You will want to talk to both people who had the surgery recently and those who had it years ago. Ask to see before and after pictures. You might also ask other patients to see their scars if you are curious about this. Most weight-loss surgery patients do not mind sharing this kind of information but ask respectfully and be considerate of the other person's privacy.

You might want to discuss the procedure with your primary care provider, although many general practitioners will not know much about weight-loss surgery, especially this relatively new procedure.

The Internet is a good place to research these kinds of topics, although you must be aware that everything you read on the Internet is not necessarily factual or correct information. You will want to visit the manufacturers' web sites, the sites of other surgeons and sites posted by patients. You will also find email support groups where people from all over the world discuss their experiences with weight-loss surgery.

If you are inclined, you can visit a medical library or website and search for articles about weight-loss surgery published in the medical literature. Most libraries will have a librarian who can help you with this.

You might choose to read other books about weight-loss surgery. It would be a good idea to read the patient instruction book that the manufacturer provides. As you do your research, keep a list of questions and try to get these answered by your doctor or other patients before surgery.

CHAPTER 4

▼

BENEFITS AND RISKS

WHAT ARE THE POTENTIAL BENEFITS OF WEIGHT-LOSS SURGERY?

Losing weight will definitely change your life and the changes are likely to be quite dramatic. No one can predict exactly what these changes will be for you. Some of the benefits you might enjoy are:

Improved physical status

Generally, after losing weight people report improvements in their physical status such as lower blood pressure, lower blood sugar, and less shortness of breath. People also report having more energy, fewer aches and pains and improved sleeping. A loss of as little as 20 pounds can result in improved mobility.

Improved psychological status

People who have lost significant amounts of weight report feeling less depressed, improved self-esteem, improved social relationships, more confidence and realistic hope for the future.

Relationships

Changes in relationships, including those with family, love relationships, friends and co-workers will occur. In general, these changes are positive and exciting. They are also demanding and occasionally may upset loved ones. Sometimes patients have trouble with a spouse's jealousy or discomfort when they become more attractive or independent.

A stable relationship is generally not harmed by weight loss and many people report their relationships are enhanced after losing weight. However, unstable relationships are seldom improved when one person decides to change dramatically. Sometimes wanting to lose weight is a sign that you also want to change your living situation, your friends or your partner. If there are fundamental difficulties with a relationship they often come to the surface after weight-loss surgery.

Self-esteem and body image

People who lose weight undergo incredible changes in how they see and feel about their bodies. Losing lots of weight creates drastic changes in body size, appearance, and related areas such as clothing choices and feelings of being attractive and sexy. Most people report increased feelings of confidence and self-esteem. Accepting a normal body image is sometimes a major challenge for weight-loss surgery patients. People who have lost lots of weight sometimes still "feel fat" at normal body weight. Some people have difficulties accepting an accurate perception of their own body size. There may be excessive fears about gaining weight back. A period of adjustment may be necessary to accept the new reality. For most people eventually the new body image becomes comfortable and reliable.

BECCA'S STORY

I started out my journey towards banded life at 5'8" tall and 496 pounds. In 18 months, I have lost 132 pounds. A whole person, some might say. I am still a work in progress, but even after losing only part of my excess weight, I have gained a whole new level of understanding of who I am and where I am destined to go in life.

Being banded not only changed my way of eating it also changed my outlook. Before I never thought that I had anything that I could contribute, since I was of the mindset that people could not (would not) see beyond my physical size. I have since learned that the qualities that I denied in myself are coming back to the surface and have found new outlets in the things that I like to do.

I may not be the best with words to express what the band has done for me, but I feel that I have regained my life, a longer, healthier life with my husband.

HOW RISKY IS GASTRIC BANDING?

Every surgery carries with it the possibility of complications. These can range from minor annoyances to major problems and even death. Each person must weigh the benefits of the surgery against the risks of complications and the risks of not having surgery. Published reports indicate that there are fewer risks from laparoscopic adjustable gastric banding surgery than from other surgical treatments for obesity.

GENERAL SURGICAL RISKS

Obesity, age and other diseases increase your risks from any surgery. There are risks that come with anesthesia and the various medications that are used in the surgical procedure.

Death is a possibility with any surgery, although death from laparoscopic adjustable gastric banding is extremely rare. Currently the chances of death from the gastric banding are estimated to be one death in 500 surgeries (0.2%).

You could have a heart attack, stroke or allergic reaction during any surgery.

An infection might occur after any surgery.

Most post-op infections can be controlled with antibiotics. If you experience any fever, chills, undue tenderness, pain, drainage, pus or increased warmth around the surgical sites, you will need to let your surgeon know immediately.

The antibiotics may not work and in some cases infection can become extremely serious and life threatening. However, this is not common.

The stomach, liver, spleen, intestines or another organ might accidentally be perforated during surgery. A blood vessel or nerve could be damaged during the surgery. You might require additional surgery to repair this kind of damage should it occur.

You might have a blood clot during or after surgery, which could cause additional problems or require additional medications or surgery. Conversely you might have uncontrolled bleeding during surgery. If you have a tendency towards either of these problems or if these problems occur your surgeon can give you medications to prevent and treat them.

Sometimes wounds rupture or fail to heal after surgery or require prolonged healing time.

COMPLICATIONS OF GASTRIC BANDING

The band may slip or migrate, or the stomach can slip. This is more likely if it is not properly sutured in place, if an infection develops or if the balloon is filled with too much fluid too soon. Patients who chronically over eat and vomit too frequently are at higher risk for slippage. Sometimes the band slips even when everything is done right.

There may be port problems. The injection port may slip or become dislocated. The tubing may become disconnected. You might have a reaction to having a foreign object implanted in your body. Although these things happen rarely you should be aware of the possibility of these problems.

When injecting into the port there is a slight risk that the silicone tubing might be punctured, causing it to leak. If this happens, the port can be replaced or the tubing repaired in a local surgery.

Some people may have unpredictable stomach swelling after an adjustment. Generally this will resolve after a few days of feeling too tight but in some cases fluid will have to be removed from the band in order to get the swelling to go down.

Leakage might occur from either the band's balloon, from the port or from the tubing between the port and the balloon. This might require a second operation. In case of leaking, the band, port or tubing can usually be replaced with a new part.

The pouch above the balloon may become enlarged so that eating is not as restricted as it should be. Conversely the opening between the upper and lower stomach might become blocked. Blockage can be caused by food, swelling, improper placement of the band, over inflation of the balloon, band or stomach slippage, stomach pouch twisting or stomach pouch enlargement. While these problems are rare, you should know that they are possible.

The esophagus can become enlarged or dilated after surgery. This might be due to improper placement of the band, stoma obstruction, binge eating, excessive vomiting or the band being over-inflated.

The esophagus or stomach can become swollen after surgery. This might require an additional hospital stay, several days of nothing to eat and intravenous fluids until the swelling goes down. In very rare cases, band removal is necessary.

The risk of an operation failing always exists, even if none of the above-mentioned complications occur. Sometimes, even though the surgery was performed correctly, a person can fail to lose weight. Generally this is due to behavioral problems like drinking too many high-calorie liquids, emotional eating and grazing on high-calorie foods all day long. But even when a person tries to eat according to the post-op plan, he or she may not lose enough to be considered a success. Most people believe you have to lose at least 50% of your excess body weight to be considered successful. You can still have dramatic health improvements with less weight loss but you wouldn't technically be considered successful.

The patient needs to understand the possibility of reoperation is an integral part of the overall surgical management of obesity. Reoperations should be considered technical measures that are sometimes necessary. The rate of reoperations is low and the possible necessity to reoperate must not be considered a failure of the surgery. Problems can usually be corrected and patients are generally rapidly back on track after a reoperation.

OTHER COMPLICATIONS

There is a risk of stomach ulcers, gastritis (stomach irritation), heartburn, bloating, trouble swallowing, dehydration, constipation and gastroesophageal reflux after adjustable gastric banding. Many of these complications can be managed with changing your diet or taking medications but some may necessitate releasing or removing the band if they become serious.

There have been some rare instances of the band eroding the wall of the stomach. This could happen right after surgery or years later. This means the stomach tissue actually grows around the band and the band ends up on the inside of the stomach rather than on the outside where it was originally placed. If this happens the band will probably need to be removed. It may be possible to place another gastric band or have another weight-loss surgery if this happens.

Complications could reduce the amount of weight lost or lead to weight regain.

Some patients have prolonged nausea and vomiting. If you have this you should report it to your surgeon immediately. Most of the time nausea and vomiting can be controlled with medications.

You can develop gallstones after rapid weight loss. This can make it necessary to remove your gall bladder. This is less likely with the gastric banding than with other forms of weight-loss surgery because the rate of weight loss is slow but it is a possibility with any form of weight loss, even dieting. There are pills you can take to prevent the development of gallstones if you are concerned about this.

If you lose weight too quickly you may have symptoms of malnutrition, anemia, low protein levels or other problems. Low vitamin, iron, or calcium levels can also occur. You may need to take supplements if you have problems getting sufficient nutrition after surgery. This is very rare with the gastric band since everything you eat will be digested normally but can occur if you are not eating enough or not eating the right foods.

If complications occur you may need to stay in the hospital longer or return to the hospital later.

If you have an existing problem, such as diabetes, you may need to take other precautions during and after surgery. Because your food intake will change, your medication needs might be affected and you will need to monitor your blood sugar closely and work with a diabetes specialist after surgery. People who take blood pressure medications also will need to have their blood pressure monitored and work with their health care provider, because their need for medication may decrease with their weight loss.

This book should not be considered a complete list of all the complications that can occur. It is for general information only and is not meant to replace professional medical advice. You need to discuss the possible complications with your surgeon and read the consent form for surgery carefully.

There may be other rare, unspecified complications. There are no guarantees that any weight-loss surgery will work without fault for the rest of your life. However, failures are rare. In most patients the adjustable gastric band will work well and provide excellent long-term weight loss.

CHAPTER 5

▼

DEALING WITH OTHERS

SHOULD I TELL MY FRIENDS AND FAMILY ABOUT THIS?

The decision about whether or not to tell close friends and family that you are having or have had weight-loss surgery is a very personal one. Some people choose not to tell because they do not like the feeling of being watched or supervised. Sometimes others will offer too much unsolicited advice about how one should eat or exercise after weight-loss surgery. Some people feel that others put too much pressure on them to lose weight after the operation. Others feel they need the support of those close to them and will discuss every aspect of the surgery in great detail with family, friends, and co-workers. It is important to remember that once you tell someone about your surgery, you cannot "untell" it.

There is no one right answer. However, you should be aware that some people may not react positively to the announcement that you have had or are having weight-loss surgery. Many will misunderstand, some will fear for your health and safety and some will be jealous. You may also have people in your life that will miss you as one of their eating buddies or feel that you are no longer one of them because you have changed. People treat you differently when you have a smaller body size, and you will need to prepare yourself for these changes.

Sometimes relationships or marriages break up when one partner changes dramatically. Many times these were relationships that were not too stable to begin with, and the desire to change drastically by losing weight is a symptom of unhappiness or the desire to seek other partners. Occasionally people who have not thought of themselves as sexual beings because of their excess weight will have trouble handling their sexuality when they are thinner. They may act out these feelings by flirting or having affairs that damage their relationships. If you think or suspect that you may have these kinds of problems as you lose weight it would be a good idea to discuss these issues with your partner or a qualified counselor.

You also may find people who accuse you of "taking the easy way out." Of course weight-loss surgery is not all that "easy." The important thing is that it is a way out.

MY FAMILY AND FRIENDS ARE NOT SUPPORTIVE

It can be very challenging to deal with people around you who seem to be to hampering, hurting or subverting your goals of achieving and maintaining a healthy body weight. Some examples of ways in which people might do this are:

- People may withdraw or no longer share their friendship with you

- Partners may become jealous and question your activities or accuse you of flirtations or affairs

- Partners may start affairs of their own while you are losing weight

- Partners might not approve or forbid you to pursue opportunities that you might have as a result of weight loss, such as working outside the home or returning to school

Sometimes losing weight creates relationship problems that you think weight regain would solve. If this happens it can be a very emotionally hurtful time. It helps to understand why this might occur.

Family therapists believe that your close friends and family are a powerful emotional system. Each person in your sphere has a place of power and attachment determined by the needs of the group or couple. Each member works to maintain their position so as to protect the cohesiveness of the group. When one person makes a drastic change, like losing a significant amount of weight, it upsets the balance of power and attachment. To maintain balance the other members must either change or resist the change in hopes of re-establishing the former familiar dynamic of power and attachment. If the other members do not change with the individual, or if they are unsuccessful in resisting the change, the system will break down. Marriages are especially vulnerable to breakdown when one partner changes and the other does not.

Successful weight loss patients experience change not only in their weight, but also in their health, self-esteem, confidence and personality, as well as increased participation in social, education and career opportunities. Most weight-loss surgery patients feel enriched by the change. When friends, spouses and family members experience the change as positive and adjust to it, relationships are often enhanced. Everyone feels they benefit from the change that the patient initiated.

When friends, spouses, and family members are disturbed or threatened by the change, they may feel they will lose their position of power or attachment and will resist the change by trying to sabotage it.

Some of the tactics of sabotage are fear, obligation and guilt. These are powerful forms of manipulation that directly or indirectly threaten punishment. They are ways of saying "if you do not do what I want, you will suffer." When confronted with these tactics, the weight-loss surgery patient faces a terrible dilemma: to pursue the change and jeopardize the relationship or sacrifice the change to protect it. Some people will tell you that there ought not to be a dilemma—your health and welfare are more important than any relationship, and if the relationship cannot adjust it should end. However, this ignores the powerful psychological, social, economic, ethical and religious importance of relationships. Furthermore, as the weight-loss surgery patients are the ones to decide whether to have surgery or not, they are also the ones to decide whether to stay in a given relationship or not.

Rather than discounting the dilemma, it is important to accept it and deal with it. One suggestion is to include potential saboteurs in the treatment process. Have your close friends or family attend a pre- or post-surgical consultation, a surgical educational session or a support group meeting. Discuss relationship benefits and stressors that you expect or experience from the weight loss. If necessary, get additional help such as discussing issues either on your own or together with a therapist or counselor.

For the best chance of success you cannot ignore the influence that your friends and family have upon your surgical outcome. It is best to address this early in the process.

HOW DO I GO ABOUT DEALING WITH THE HEALTH INSURANCE COMPANY?

Some insurance companies will cover weight-loss surgery, however, many do not and each insurance policy differs. Most surgeons will have an insurance specialist in their office that will help you work with your insurance carrier and submit all the required information to expedite their approval process. Be sure you know in advance what your insurance company is willing to cover.

If your insurance company will not pay for the cost of the surgery, you still have the option of paying for the surgery yourself. Yes, surgery is expensive, but you have to weigh the possible benefits against the costs.

TONI'S STORY

The realization that I had to do something came one day at the post office in November 2002. I opened a letter from a friend I had seen at a wedding back in April of 2002. Inside were some photos from that wedding. As I looked at them I began to cry in the post office. There I was at 258 pounds, looking so awful I was sorry I had attended.

As I drove 200 miles to attend a business meeting I couldn't think of anything else other than I had to do something. I called my mother and asked her to call a family friend who is a nurse practitioner for suggestions. She mentioned something about a surgery where they put a band around your stomach so you eat less. I immediately began searching the Internet for information on adjustable gastric banding. Before the week was out, I had a lot of information. I called the surgical group.

Before the month was out I had attended an information seminar and met the surgeon. I listed my weight as 248 on my paperwork. They said my ideal weight should be 137 so I was 111 pounds overweight. I said I would like to weigh less than when I got married at 170 pounds. The day I reach 170 I am going to get all fixed up, do my hair, put on make-up, and put on my wedding dress. That was the only day I felt totally beautiful and I want to have that feeling again.

The struggle began when I heard that my insurance would not cover the procedure. I was very lucky in that I work for the Federal Government and have several choices for insurance coverage and open season was within the next few weeks.

I changed insurance and made an appointment for a pre-surgery consult. After two visits my insurance request for approval was denied. The staff at the doctor's office filed my appeal letter, which included letters of support from three of my regular medical providers. Also, they included 12 years of medical records. My surgery was approved on appeal May 13. My surgery was scheduled for July 11. I was so excited I could hardly believe it.

I couldn't walk or exercise without my chest and knees hurting. I felt bad both mentally and physically. I started to feel better after losing the first 10 pounds.

Less than 8 months after having surgery I had lost the 78 pounds needed to fit into my wedding dress again. I once again feel totally beautiful. I'd actually like to lose a few more pounds and get down to maybe 150 but now I know it will happen. This surgery saved my life. I had been so miserable. Losing weight doesn't solve all your problems, but it has made me a happier person to know that I have control over my eating.

CHAPTER 6

▼

HAVING SURGERY AND THE FIRST FEW WEEKS

IS THERE ANYTHING I SHOULD DO BEFORE SURGERY?

Some surgeons will ask you to lose weight before surgery. You may be asked to go on a diet or meal plan or to consume only liquids for two or three weeks before the surgery. The purpose of this is to make your liver smaller, therefore making the surgery easier. There isn't much concrete evidence that dieting before surgery actually shrinks the liver, however many surgeons have observed this in their practice and believe it to be true. If your surgeon asks you to do this, it would be a good idea to try to comply.

In general, try to comply with everything your surgeon requests. Different combinations work better for different surgeons. The suggestions in this book should not be used as an excuse for not following your own doctors' recommendations.

HOW LONG DO I HAVE TO STAY IN THE HOSPITAL?

Your surgeon will have a policy about how long you should stay in the hospital. Most people leave the hospital one to three days. If you have any complications such as bleeding, swelling or infection you may have to stay longer. In some surgical centers, adjustable gastric banding is being performed as an outpatient surgery. You would have the surgery early in the morning and be able to leave in the afternoon the same day.

WHAT TESTS ARE ASSOCIATED WITH GASTRIC BANDING?

You will need to ask your surgeon about what tests he recommends. General tests such as those performed before any surgery might include blood tests, a urinalysis, a chest x-ray or an electrocardiogram. Your surgeon will either perform a complete physical exam and medical history or want a copy of these from another health care provider.

You may need to have your gastrointestinal tract examined with x-rays or a fluoroscope before or after the surgery. A fluoroscope is just a video form of x-rays. You may be asked to swallow a liquid like barium that can be seen moving into your stomach on a TV screen as you swallow. After surgery these tests can help your health care team know that the band is in the right place and functioning well. You may need to have this fluoroscopy or x-rays repeated when your band is being filled or if you have problems.

If you took phen-fen diet pills the anesthesiologist may want you to have an echocardiogram to be sure your heart valves were not damaged by this medication. If you have had this done already, a copy of the report may be enough.

Many obese people have undiagnosed sleep apnea. Sleep apnea is a serious disease that causes you to stop breathing while you are sleeping. If your doctors feel this might be a problem for you they will want you to get a sleep study. It is important to know this before giving anesthesia to someone with sleep apnea. If you already know you have this and are using a continuous positive airway pressure (C-PAP) machine to help your breathing during sleep, you may be asked to bring your machine with you to the hospital so the nurses can apply it while you are sleeping after surgery.

If you have diabetes it will be important to be in good control before undergoing an elective surgery. Some of the blood tests performed will assess your degree of diabetes control.

WHAT IS THE IMMEDIATE POST-OP RECOVERY PERIOD LIKE?

Your surgeon will give you post-op instructions.

For the first few days after surgery you may be a bit sore. You should take it easy and plan to get plenty of rest but at the same time you should remain active and get up and walk around several times a day, taking deep breaths. This gets your blood circulating and helps prevent breathing problems like pneumonia and blood clots that can occur if you are too inactive after surgery.

Most surgeons recommend that you stay on liquids for several days to a few weeks after gastric banding. You will need to take very small sips of liquids very gradually at first. Drinking too much or too fast may cause you to have nausea and vomiting. If you have trouble with this you may need to ask your doctor for medication to control nausea until your stomach settles down. Avoid extremely cold beverages until you can sip them gradually.

The length of time that you need to stay on the liquids varies from surgeon to surgeon so you will have to ask for specific instructions about when you can have thicker liquids and when you can return to eating regular food.

The liquid phase is very important in order to allow the stomach to heal and for the band to seat properly in place. There are a few sutures holding the band in place that must not be disturbed until they heal. Eating too much too soon is associated with band slippage especially if you eat things that might cause you to vomit or things that would cause your stomach to churn while trying to digest them. Stick to the liquids for as long as your doctor requires.

This liquid phase is not a weight-loss phase. It is a time for healing and allowing the stomach to recover from surgery and to adapt to the presence of the band. Many people lose weight during the liquid phase but some do not begin to lose much weight until after the first adjustment. If this happens to you all you need to do is be patient. Weight loss will occur. It just takes time and it doesn't always start right away. Generally the first adjustment is not done until four to eight weeks after surgery, and if you are losing weight well you may not need an adjustment even then.

WHY CAN'T I SMOKE AFTER SURGERY?

Smoking can interfere with healing after surgery. Smoking constricts blood vessels and decreases blood flow all over the body. Even more important, the carbon monoxide in cigarette smoke greatly reduces the blood's ability to carry oxygen that is essential for wound healing.

If you smoke after surgery and have a bout of hard coughing you could cause internal bleeding. For these reasons some doctors will advise you to give up smoking before surgery. If you are having surgery to improve your looks and well being it makes little sense to jeopardize the results by failing to forego smoking for several weeks. If you are willing to quit permanently this may be an excellent time to do so.

WHEN CAN I RETURN TO WORK?

This depends on the type of work you do and the type of surgery you have. Ask your doctor for a specific recommendation about returning to work. Someone with a desk job can usually return to work a few days after the basic laparoscopic adjustable gastric band. If you have a strenuous job or a job that requires heavy lifting you may need to be off work or on light duty for a couple weeks. If you have a more extensive surgery you will be off work longer.

If you don't want people at your work to know you had weight-loss surgery you doctor can give you a generic note that does not specify the type of surgery you had. You are not required to disclose your personal medical history to your employer. If they ask you can say it's personal, or that you would rather not discuss it.

WHAT CAN I HAVE DURING THE LIQUID PHASE OF THE POST-OP DIET?

You should do your best to follow the instructions given to you by your particular surgeon. The purpose of this special diet is to allow the stitches in and around your stomach to completely heal and for the band to become seated in the right position, not to lose weight. Consuming only liquids for a few weeks after surgery avoids stretching the new pouch. It is very important not to stress or stretch the newly created upper pouch during the healing phase. You should not be eating things that would cause your stomach to churn. Stick to liquids that easily run into the lower portion of the stomach.

Right after surgery you may have some tiny sips of water or suck on ice chips. Gradually, in several hours or the day after surgery you will be allowed to have more fluids, but you should sip small amounts at a time. Gulping these liquids or drinking too much at one time can cause nausea and vomiting, which you want to avoid as much as possible.

It is common to have a period of a few days to several weeks where you will be asked to consume liquids only. This will gradually be increased from clear liquids to full liquids. Clear liquids are those you can see through like water, sugar free juice, tea, clear broth and the like. Full liquids include non-fat milk, creamed soups, pudding, low-fat yogurt, pureed fruit and instant breakfast or protein drinks. Liquids are things that you can get through a straw. You will be allowed to gradually increase your diet to include soft foods and then eventually move to regular foods. Soft foods are those things you can eat without teeth. Once you move to regular food you will have to chew your food well.

CLEAR LIQUID DIET

The clear liquid diet is a temporary diet. The clear liquid diet helps to keep you hydrated (body fluids, salts, and minerals) and helps to get the body used to food after surgery. The clear liquid diet is easy to digest and does not leave much residue in the stomach and intestines.

Liquids that you can see through at room temperature are considered clear liquids. This includes clear juices, broths, ices, and gelatin. The table below will help you with your choices.

	Choose these foods/beverages	Do not eat these foods/beverages
Fruits/Juices	Ice chips, water, flavored water, clear fruit juices without pulp such as apple juice, grape juice, and cranberry juice, Gatorade. Use low-sugar versions.	Nectars, canned, fresh, or frozen fruits. Do not use carbonated or sweetened beverages.
Soups	Broth, bouillon, fat free consommé	Cream soups, soups with vegetables, noodles, rice, meat, or other chunks of food in them.
Beverages	Coffee, tea, herbal teas (hot or cold), sugar free Kool-Aid, Crystal Light, water.	All others
Sweets & Desserts	Fruit ices (without chunks of fruit), plain gelatin, popsicles made from clear juices.	All others
Vegetables	None	All
Milk & Dairy Products	None	All
Bread, cereals, and grain products	None	All
Meat, chicken, fish, and meat substitutes (nuts, tofu etc)	None	All
Oils, butter, margarine	None	All

Sample Clear Liquid Diet	
Breakfast:	Hot tea with lemon juice (no pulp); low sugar apple juice; gelatin
Lunch:	Hot tea with lemon (no pulp); low sugar grape juice; fruit ice; consommé
Snack:	Fruit juice (apple, cranberry, or grape); gelatin
Dinner:	Hot tea with lemon (no pulp); apple juice; consommé; fruit ice

FULL LIQUID DIET

The full liquid diet is a temporary diet. The full liquid diet helps to keep your body hydrated (body fluids, salts, and minerals) and helps to get the body used to food after surgery. The full liquid is a temporary transition phase between clear liquids and soft foods. The full liquid diet is easy to digest and does not leave much residue in the stomach and intestines. You can still have all the things on the clear liquid diet too.

If you have lactose intolerance or have trouble digesting milk products you can use soy or rice milk instead of cow's milk or take Lactaid. Lactaid is a dietary supplement that helps to break down milk sugar.

	Choose these foods/beverages	Do not eat these foods/beverages
Fruits/Juices	Fruit juices without pulp such as apple juice, grape juice, cranberry juice, and nectars. Use low sugar versions.	Canned, fresh, or frozen fruits.
Soups	Broth, bouillon, fat free consommé, or strained cream soups. Tomato soup made with milk or water.	Soups with vegetables, noodles, rice, meat, or other chunks of food in them. Strain these items from the soup and blend them or just have the broth
Beverages	Coffee, tea (hot or cold), sugar free Kool-Aid, Crystal Light, Gatorade, or water	All others
Sweets & Desserts	Fruit ices (without chunks of fruit), plain gelatin, popsicles made from sugar-free juices, custards, and pudding	All others
Vegetables	None	All others
Milk and dairy products	Non-fat milk, yogurt, Carnation Instant Breakfast	Ice cream
Meat, chicken, fish, and meat substitutes (nuts, tofu etc)	None	All
Oils, butter, & margarine	None	All

Sample Full Liquid Diet	
Breakfast	Hot tea with lemon or non-fat milk; yogurt
Lunch	Hot tea with lemon; strained cream of potato soup; non-fat milk
Snack	Low sugar fruit juice (apple, cranberry, or grape)
Dinner	Hot tea with lemon or non-fat milk; strained or blended cream of asparagus soup; pudding

SOFT DIET

The soft diet serves as a transition from liquids to a regular diet for individuals who are recovering from surgery. It can ease difficulty in swallowing and relieve mild intestinal or stomach discomfort. You can still have all the things on the clear liquid and full liquid diet, too.

The soft diet limits or eliminates foods that are hard to chew and swallow, such as raw fruits and vegetables, chewy breads, and tough meats. Fried, greasy foods and highly seasoned or spicy foods are not included. You should practice chewing your food well even though you may not have to.

You can soften foods by cooking or mashing. Household tools and machines such as a blender, food processor, meat grinder, or knife, can make foods easier to chew and swallow. Canned or soft-cooked fruits and vegetables may be used in place of raw or dry varieties. Refined cereals are recommended over coarse, whole-grain types. Moist, tender meats, fish, and poultry are permitted.

	Choose these foods/beverages	Do not eat these foods/beverages
Beverages	All	None
Soups	Mildly seasoned broth, bouillon, or cream soup; strained vegetable soup.	Bean, gumbo, split pea, or onion soup; chunky soups or chowders.
Meat, chicken, fish, and meat substitutes (nuts, tofu etc)	Any moist, tender meat. Fish, or poultry (lamb, veal, chicken, turkey, tender beef, liver, strewed pork); soft cooked eggs, poached eggs, soft boiled eggs. Use marinade, stews or a pressure cooker to tenderize.	Fried chicken or fish; fish with bones; shellfish; fried, salted, or smoked meats; sausage; cold cuts; fried eggs; dried beans; nuts and seeds.
Dairy	All low-fat milk products, smooth yogurt, mild flavored cheese, cottage cheese.	Avoid milk if lactose intolerant; yogurt with nuts or seeds; sharp or strong cheeses; cheeses with whole seeds or spices.
Fruits	Mashed, cooked, or canned fruit; soft fresh banana; applesauce, low sugar fruit juice.	All raw fruit (except banana); dried fruit (dates, raisins); coconut.
Vegetables	Soft-cooked or canned vegetables; tomatoes; potatoes (mashed, baked, boiled, or creamed).	Whole kernel corn, raw vegetables, fried vegetables, French fries, hash browns.
Grains	Refined, cooked or ready-to-eat cereal; crackers. Oatmeal, cream of wheat, grits.	Whole-grain breads and cereals (bran rye with seeds, or whole wheat); breads or rolls with coconut, raisins, nuts, or seeds.
Fats	Butter, margarine; mild salsas; low-fat dressing; low-fat mayonnaise; low-fat sour cream; vegetable oil.	Spicy salad dressings; fried foods.
Desserts & Sweets	Smooth ice milk or frozen yogurt; sherbet; fruit ices; custards; puddings.	Desserts or candy made with dried fruits, nuts, or coconut; candied fruit; peanut brittle; ice cream.
Seasonings	Ketchup; tomato or white spices; soy sauce; chopped or ground leaf herbs.	Garlic; horseradish; chili powder; whole or seed herbs and spices; barbeque or Cajun seasonings.

Sample Soft Diet	
Breakfast	Low-sugar juice, runny oatmeal or other cooked cereal, whole-wheat crackers, soft-boiled or poached eggs, soft banana, and non-fat milk.
Lunch	Soft white fish, crackers, creamed broccoli flowerets, cottage cheese.
Dinner	Cream of potato soup, boneless marinated chicken breast, grilled zucchini, crackers, creamed vegetable or sweet potato without skin, soft fruit, sugar-free pudding, non-fat milk.

After 4 to 6 weeks you can gradually transition to regular foods. Cut food into small pieces, eat slowly and chew well. Stop eating at the first hint of fullness. Do not drink liquids with your foods. Don't forget to take your daily vitamin supplement.

WHY CAN'T I HAVE CARBONATED BEVERAGES AFTER SURGERY?

Some surgeons feel that carbonated beverages might contribute to stretching the upper stomach pouch after surgery. Carbonated beverages tend to release their gases when they warm up inside the body. The can make you feel full and cause burping and discomfort. Therefore they should be avoided.

Some band patients will try to continue drinking these beverages after they go flat. Ways to make soda pop lose its carbonation include leaving an open can or bottle in the refrigerator over night, stirring or shaking the container to release the bubbles, pouring the beverage over ice, or adding a little artificial sweetener. If you try all these things chances are you will find that carbonated beverages don't taste all that good and they are not worth the trouble. They still may contain enough gas to cause your pouch to stretch even when they taste flat.

WHAT CAN I HAVE DURING THE SOFT FOODS PHASE OF THE POST-OP DIET?

Once again, most likely your surgeon will have given you specific instructions about this. You should do your best to follow the instructions given to you by your particular surgeon. The soft foods phase usually begins two to four weeks after surgery and can last for two to four weeks.

During this phase (which I like to call slush and mush) you can have all the things that you had during the liquid phase plus some creamier soups. You can begin to add moist blended meat like beef, chicken and veal or fish to your diet. Many types of meat can be blended with liquids such as gravy, stock, soup, vegetable juice or white sauce. Casseroles can also be blended with added liquids.

Smoothies made with fresh fruits, yogurt, and crushed ice are also suitable for this period. Moist cereals such as oatmeal, cream of wheat or porridge can be made suitable with extra water or milk.

Some people eat baby food or toddler meals from a jar during the slush and mush phase. They are the right consistency, but most adults find baby food is really bland and doesn't taste very good.

You will need to take very small bites and chew all of your food extremely well. If you do not follow this precaution you may have vomiting, stomach irritation, swelling or obstruction. Many people have trouble with foods such as bread, rice and fibrous vegetables and you will want to avoid these in the early weeks.

The bad thing about the slush and mush phase is that it teaches you that these soft foods that can be fairly high in calories go down easily. This is not a good lesson to learn and you should move from the slush and mush to regular food as soon as your stomach is healed. Regular food will stay in the pouch longer and make you feel full and satisfied. The goal of banding is to be able to eat small quantities of real food, not to switch to a pureed diet.

Chapter 7

▼

Adjusting the Adjustable Gastric Band

What is a Band Adjustment?

An adjustment is adding fluid to the balloon around your stomach. This tightens the band and makes the opening between the upper and lower portions of the stomach smaller so less food and fluid will go through. Adjustments are also called "fills" or inflations.

An adjustment can also refer to un-filling. Sometimes when the band is too tight, fluid needs to be removed.

Generally most people require three to five adjustments during the first year. Most bariatric practices do adjustments on an as needed basis. Whenever you stop losing weight for three weeks you should contact your surgeon's office about a possible adjustment.

How is an Adjustment Done?

Sometimes adjustments are done in an outpatient clinic or office. Sometimes they are carried out in an X-ray department under fluoroscopy. Fluoroscopy is just a form of moving X-ray. The picture shows up on a monitor where the radiologist or another doctor can watch it. If you are having X-rays you may be asked not to take anything by mouth for several hours before the X-ray. It would be very hard to see what is going on if your stomach were full of food at the time of the X-ray.

When X-rays are used the exact position of the band and the degree of tightness can be ascertained by having you drink a special liquid that shows up on the screen or film.

X-rays are not necessarily required and your doctor may be comfortable adding (or removing fluid) from your band without the additional time, expense, and exposure to radiation that you would get if you needed an X-ray. If your port is very deep or if it ends up tilted, or is otherwise difficult to access it may be necessary to use the fluoroscope to locate the port.

To do the adjustment a fine needle is passed through the skin into the port to add or remove saline. Local anesthesia may or may not be needed. Most people find adjustments don't hurt much. They are similar to getting your blood drawn. You will probably be lying down. The doctor may ask you to raise your head or feet to contract the abdominal muscles and make the port easier to feel. Sometimes adjustments can be done while sitting or standing. The adjustment process normally takes only a few minutes.

You will want to try drinking some water before leaving the X-ray department or the office. This is not a guarantee that your fill level is correct, but if the water does not go down it is quite likely that you are too tight and you can save yourself a second trip to have fluid removed by testing this right after the adjustment. Although water is probably available, some patients bring a water bottle with them to the adjustment appointment.

You doctor may ask you not to eat or drink for several hours before an adjustment. It's also a good idea to sip fluids slowly and gradually reintroduce eating solid foods for the first several hours or for a day or so after an adjustment. Usually you will feel increased restriction when you first try to eat after a new adjustment. Sometimes the stomach may swell or get a bit irritated from an adjustment. However, this should pass in a few days and you should be able to take in small amounts of food. You should always be able to take in sufficient fluid. You may experience increased vomiting until you learn to eat with your new level of restriction. If you experience prolonged vomiting (more than once or twice) or you cannot drink fluids or eat after a fill then you may be too tight and you may need to go back and have some fluid let out.

You need to call your doctor immediately if you are unable to take in sufficient fluids and are having signs of dehydration. These would include a very dry mouth, decreased urination and dark and strong urine. Rapid weight loss, feeling dizzy, having sunken eyes and a rapid pulse and rapid breathing are late signs of dehydration. You should not wait that long to contact your health care provider.

WHEN DO I HAVE THE FIRST ADJUSTMENT?

The average time for a first adjustment is about four to eight weeks after surgery. If you are losing weight at a rate of one to two pounds a week without an adjustment your surgeon may want you to wait until your weight loss stops or slows before adjusting the band. There is no advantage to having the band any tighter than it needs to be.

Some surgeons fill the band a bit at the time of surgery. If you had this done you may need to wait longer for a first adjustment.

HOW MANY ADJUSTMENTS ARE NEEDED?

Your surgeon will give you instructions about adjustments. On average three to five adjustments are done spaced apart about every month or two during the first year. If you are monitoring your weight loss you will know when you need another adjustment because your weight loss will stop or slow. When you have weighed the same for three or four weeks in a row, it is time to contact your surgeon about an adjustment.

You cannot tell that you need an adjustment by how much you are eating. The amount you can eat will normally vary quite a bit from day to day. Weigh yourself once a week and use that as your guide.

HOW DO I KNOW IF I NEED TO HAVE FLUID LET OUT?

If you are unable to swallow your saliva, unable to drink an adequate amount of fluid, or unable to eat solid food you may have an obstruction or your band may be too tight. If this goes on for more than a few hours you will become seriously dehydrated. You may even faint from severe dehydration. You need to call your health care provider whenever you experience these symptoms.

Frequent heartburn, belching, and regurgitation can be signs that your band is too tight. If you are having reflux at night more than once a week you should let your health care provider know. Reflux is when food and fluids come into your mouth and nose when you lie down. You may wake up coughing from these symptoms. Some people even have reflux during the day while sitting or standing.

Other signs that your band might be too tight include difficulty swallowing. It may be hard to get food down even when it is well-chewed. If you can only eat soft foods your band may be too tight.

In some people a tight band can also cause symptoms that resemble other respiratory conditions, such as sore throat, wheezing, chronic coughing, and hoarseness.

HOW CAN I TELL IF I AM PERFECTLY ADJUSTED?

If you are losing one or two pounds per week and you are eating well and vomiting rarely you are probably perfectly adjusted. If you are not losing one or two pounds per week you may need to make one of the following adjustments.

Questions to determine if you need an eating adjustment

- Are you eating 60 grams of protein a day?
- Are you eating 25 grams of fiber?
- Are you avoiding all liquid calories? (except two servings of non-fat milk)
  - Soup can be sign of "soft calorie syndrome"
  - Alcohol contains a lot of calories—7 calories per gram
    - It's also a stomach irritant
  - Fruit juice is just sugar water
- Are you making healthy food choices from a wide variety of foods?
- Are you avoiding soft foods?
  - You can't just eat what's easy
  - Cheese and peanut butter are glorified fats (read the labels)
- Are you drinking six to eight glasses of water a day between meals?
- Are you eating too much junk?
  - Chips, chocolate, nuts, ice cream, cookies and other highly processed junk foods are too calorie dense to be regular parts of a healthy diet. But don't avoid them completely to the point where you feel deprived
  - Stay out of fast food places (alcoholics don't hang out in bars)
- Are you getting in two servings of calcium daily?
- Do you always eat the protein first?
- Do you then eat the vegetables or fruits?

- You need three to five servings of vegetables or fruits a day
- Potatoes are NOT a vegetable
- Is your portion size appropriate?
  - Meat or fish—three ounces—the size of a deck of cards or a computer mouse
  - Vegetables1/2 cup—the size of your fist
  - Starch—if you eat the protein and the vegetables first you don't need much
    - Avoid: bread, rice, potatoes, pasta
- You might try avoiding artificial sweeteners.
  - Some people think that artificial sweeteners stimulate the appetite. They are HUNDREDS of times sweeter than sugar and they teach you to like things too sweet. There is no evidence that people who use them are any thinner than people who don't
- Avoid most diet foods
  - Real food usually tastes better
  - Real food is more satisfying than low-calorie substitutes
  - When you are only eating a tiny bit the caloric savings are not that great
  - Use a teaspoon of real butter instead of a tablespoon of diet margarine
- The body has no way to break down artificial fats (trans-fats)
  - They may go into permanent storage
  - Some people think liposuction is the only way to remove hydrolyzed fats from the body

Questions to determine if you need a behavior adjustment

- Are you eating only when you are hungry?

- If you're not sure, drink at least eight ounces of water and wait

- Are you eating three meals a day? (with maybe one or two small planned snacks)

- Are you sitting down to eat?

- Are you eating consciously?

  - No distractions, turn off the TV, put the book or newspaper away, pay attention to your food and your companions

- Are you eating slowly?

  - Put the fork down between bites

  - Take 20 to 30 minutes to finish a meal

  - Taking longer might cause the pouch to begin emptying

- Are you taking small bites?

  - Tiny spoon, chopsticks, cocktail fork

- Are you chewing well?

- Are you drinking with your meals or too soon after your meals?

  - You won't be thirsty if you are well hydrated before the meal

- Practice water loading between meals

- Are you stopping at the first sign of fullness?

  - Sometimes it's a whisper: not hungry, had enough

- Do not eat between meals. Stop grazing

- Do not eat when you are not hungry

Questions to determine if you need an activity adjustment

- Are you getting in 30 minutes of physical activity at least 3 times a week?
  - Over and above what you would do in the usual course of your day
- Could you make it four or five times a week?
- Could you make it 45 or 60 minutes?
- Are you making the most of opportunities to increase your physical activity?
  - Taking the stairs instead of the elevators or escalators
  - Walking on the escalators instead of riding
  - Parking your car further away from the entrance
  - Getting out of the car instead of using the drive-through
  - Getting off the bus one stop before your destination
  - Washing you car by hand instead of the car wash
  - Playing actively with your kids

Questions to determine if you need an attitude adjustment

- Are you committed to your weight loss journey?

- Are you totally honest with yourself about how much you are eating and exercising?

- Log your food and activity on ww.fitday.com for 3 days

- Are you using foods inappropriately to deal with emotional issues?

- Have you identified what the emotions are that drive your eating?

- Can you think of more appropriate ways to deal with those emotions?

- Are you willing to seek help from a qualified counselor?

- Are you attending and participating in support group meetings?

- Have you drummed up some support from your family and friends?

- Have you dealt with saboteurs realistically?

- Do you have realistic expectations about the weight loss journey?

- Are you still obsessing about food, weight, eating, and dieting?
  - Obsess about something else
  - Avoid perfectionism
  - Avoid all or none, black and white thinking

- Have patience with the pace of healthy weight loss

- Are you acknowledging your successes with non-food rewards?
- Have you learned how to take a compliment?
- Are you giving up diet mentality?
  - Stop weighing yourself several times a day or every day
  - Stop dieting
  - Stop depriving yourself
  - Stop defining food as "good" and "bad"
  - Stop rewarding and punishing yourself with food
- How do you feel about all the changes taking place?

Questions to determine if you need a band adjustment

- Do you feel like you are making healthy food choices in appropriate portion sizes but getting hungry between meals?
- Can you still eat white bread, fibrous vegetables, and large portions?
- Do you have to struggle to lose?
- Are you gaining weight in spite of eating right, exercising, and having a good mindset?

Questions to determine if your need your band loosened

- If there are times when you can't get fluids down?
- You are vomiting too much?
  - How much is too much?
- Do you have frequent reflux or heartburn at night?
  - Do not lie flat or bend over soon after eating
  - Do not eat late at night or just before bedtime
    Rinse your pouch with a glass of water an hour before bedtime
  - Certain foods or drinks are more likely to cause reflux:
    - Rich, spicy, fatty and fried foods
    - Chocolate
    - Caffeine
    - Alcohol
    - Some fruits and vegetables
      - Oranges, lemons, tomatoes, peppers
    - Peppermint
      - Use baking soda toothpaste instead of mint
- Carbonated drinks
- Eat slowly and do not eat big meals
- If you smoke, quit smoking
- Reduce stress
- Exercise promotes digestion
- Raise the head of your bed

- Wear loose fitting clothing around your waist
- Take estrogen containing medications in the morning
- Avoid aspirin, Aleve and ibuprofen at bedtime
- Tylenol is OK
- Take an antacid before retiring
- Try other over-the-counter heartburn medications
- See your health care provider if reflux persists

See your health care provider immediately (or call 911) if

- You have a squeezing, tightness or heaviness in your chest, especially if the discomfort spreads to your shoulder, arm or jaw or is accompanied by shortness of breath, sweating, irregular or fast heartbeat or nausea. These could be symptoms of a heart attack
- If your symptoms are triggered by exercise
- If your pain localizes to your right side, especially if you also have nausea or fever
- If you throw up vomit that looks like black sand or coffee grounds. Or if your stool is black, deep red or looks like it has tar in it. These are symptoms of bleeding and need immediate attention. (Note: Pepto-Bismol or other medications with bismuth will turn your stool black. Iron supplements can also make the stool tarry.)
- If your pain is severe

CHAPTER 8

▼

EATING AFTER GASTRIC BANDING

WHAT CAN I EAT?

By the time you are four to six weeks out from surgery your new stomach will pretty much be healed. You may have had your first fill of the balloon in the band by this time. Your doctor will have discussed what you were eating and what you should be eating now with you.

An adjustable gastric band affects the size of the opening between the upper and lower part of the stomach. When the band is tightened a smaller opening lets less food through causing greater weight loss. This also requires that patients be very careful about what they eat. With the band's balloon totally empty, the patient can eat almost normally.

You need to realize that liquids will pass through the pouch very quickly and will not make you feel full. While liquids are necessary for the healing phase, at this stage you need to avoid high-calorie liquids. Liquids such as water, broth, tea, and low-calorie vegetable juice like tomato or V-8, sugar free lemonade and coffee without sugar are all fine. It is best to get your liquid intake before meals because drinking liquid during or after meals will tend to flush food through the pouch and you will not get the sensation of fullness that you need to help you eat less.

Eating too much or swallowing food in big chunks can block the passageway between the upper and lower stomach. You can avoid this by taking small bites, chewing your food well, and eating slowly. Some people have to practice chewing well by counting 30 or 40 chews for each bite until they get use to chewing their food well. I have found that I cannot eat and talk at the same time and in addition to slowing down I have to concentrate a bit more when eating.

Rather than eating only one thing, you will find it easier to eat if you mix your textures. Take a bite of meat and then a bite of cracker or vegetable. It will go through the pouch better than eating only meat or only vegetables, which can tend to ball up and plug the stoma.

Try different cooking methods to get food textures that are band friendly. Many people find that foods cooked in a crock-pot or pressure cooker are very tender.

If you follow these cautions you can eat most things. Bread and fibrous vegetables remain a problem for most people but even those can be eaten in small amounts.

HOW DO I GO ABOUT INTRODUCING SOLID FOODS BACK INTO MY MEALS?

The biggest tip I can give you here is to take it slowly. Start with very small portions. Cut your food into small pieces. Take small bites. Chew everything really well. Eat slowly.

Gradually add new foods one at a time. Then if you have difficulty eating at a meal it will be easier to pin-point the food that may be causing you trouble. There is no food you should not try, but try things cautiously. You will soon learn what textures are best avoided.

WHAT FOODS SHOULD BE AVOIDED?

While trying to lose weight you will need to avoid foods that have a concentrated supply of calories with little nutritional value. Food with large quantities of sugar should be omitted. These are high calorie liquids, syrups, cakes, biscuits, sweets, candy, jam, marmalade, honey and the like. High-fat foods also detract from your weight-loss efforts and you should avoid chocolate, chips, pies and pastries. Alcohol is just another high-calorie liquid that will not help you with your weight-loss efforts.

You won't have to give up all these foods forever. Once you get down to your goal weight you can have small amounts of these foods once in a while, but empty-calorie foods are never going to play a big part in eating in a healthy way.

Although two servings of non-fat milk are recommended because of the calcium, you should realize that milk is relatively high in calories. An eight-ounce glass of non-fat milk contains 80 calories. While this doesn't sound like much it is eighty times the amount of calories in water, coffee, tea, and other no calorie drinks (if 80 times 0 were 80). An eight-ounce glass of 2% milk is 120 calories or a whopping 120 times the amount of calories in these other beverages. So you will need to limit your milk intake. Just because milk is allowed on the post-op diet does not mean that you can have unlimited amounts or that it is always a good choice. Some people elect not to drink milk and get their calcium from supplements or from other high calcium foods and fortified cereals.

WHAT ELSE CAN I DO TO MAXIMIZE MY CHANCES FOR WEIGHT LOSS SUCCESS?

There are many things you can do to optimize your chances of weight loss success. First drink plenty of water. Aim to take in at least six to eight glasses of water a day. Avoid drinking high-calorie liquids.

Reduce your calorie intake. In plain English, eat less. The band will help you immensely with this but you can also consciously reduce your intake by choosing to eat low fat and low calorie foods. Use lower fat foods in place of higher fat options whenever you have a choice. Minimize your intake of the saturated fats found in animal products. Watch your portion sizes. Do not risk displacing the band by over eating or causing yourself frequent vomiting.

Try to stop eating at the first sign of fullness. Anybody can stop his or her car by driving it into a brick wall. Bandsters call this the "hard stop." This is essentially what you are doing if you eat until you are stuffed or until you have a pain in your chest.

It takes more practice to learn to apply the brakes gradually before you hit the wall. You can practice doing this with your eating. This is called a "soft stop." Quit eating at the very first hint of fullness or when you are no longer hungry. You can always eat more later, if you are still hungry, but many times if you stop eating and go do something else you will forget about food for a while.

You do not have to clean your plate. If you are still having trouble doing this or are frequently tempted to take that one last bite even though you are full then you will have to measure out portions on your plate. Many banded people eat only a half a cup of food at a meal. Use smaller plates and bowls so that a half-cup of cereal actually fills a small bowl instead of looking like a tiny amount in a larger bowl.

Avoid snacking. You will take in fewer calories if you eat three small meals a day and a couple planned snacks rather than constantly grazing all day long. A planned snack might be some beef jerky, a hard-boiled egg, or two or three crackers with a little cheese in the late afternoon to keep you from getting too hungry before a late dinner.

Try to eat denser foods. Eating denser, less processed foods (such as fresh meat, fish, seafood, fruits and vegetables, whole grains, beans, lentils, and cereals will make you feel more satisfied than eating softer processed foods which pass through the band easily. Although they are often more difficult to eat after gastric banding in that you have to slow down, take smaller bites and chew more, denser foods are often packed with nutrients and flavor.

Increase your energy expenditure. That's a fancy way of saying exercise. Try to be as physically active as possible. Park further away, get off the bus one stop earlier, use the rest room that is furthest away from your office, take the stairs instead of the elevator. Every little bit helps.

Optimize your fill level. If you are not losing one to two pounds a week for 3 or more weeks then ask your doctor about adding fluid to your band.

WHAT SHOULD I BE EATING?

After you get through the first few weeks and you've had your first adjustment, you should be eating healthy meals. Most people will do fine with three small meals a day. Choose nutritious foods from all food groups. You should select fresh foods over canned or processed foods whenever possible. Avoid foods that are high in sugar or fat. If you really do not know what to eat you might want to ask your surgeon for a referral to a dietician or to see the dietician on the weight-loss surgery team for some suggestions or a meal plan.

Almost all people who are overweight have been chronic dieters and many of them know almost as much about what they should be eating as a dietician. The post-op diet is the same as many of the balanced diets you have been on before. The only reason you lose weight after banding is because your portion size is restricted and you feel full and satisfied after eating a small amount. You could get a copy of a healthy diet from the American Diabetes Association or American Heart Association or use the US Department of Agriculture's food pyramid if you truly have no idea.

For example, using the food pyramid, a typical post-op diet for a whole day might be:

- As much calorie-free, non-carbonated liquid as you want
- Two servings from the milk/yogurt group/cottage cheese
  - (eight ounces, ~90 calories, eight grams of protein)
- Four to six servings from the meat/poultry/fish/seafood/beans/eggs/ nuts group
  - (1 ounce, 55-75 calories, six to eight grams of protein)
  - (Most people eat three ounces at a meal)
- Two or three servings from the vegetable group

- (1/2 cup cooked, one cup raw, 25 calories)
- One or two servings from the fruit group
  - (one small, ~ 60 calories)
- Three to four servings from the bread/cereal, rice/pasta group
  - (five saltines or 3/4 cup cereal, ~80 calories)
- Use as little additional fat as you can get by with
- Take a multivitamin every day

The size, calories and protein numbers are estimates. This is the minimum that you should eat. Including the fats that accompany many of these foods, this diet would provide 1,000 to 1,200 calories a day. You will have to watch your protein intake to get in 60 grams of protein a day. You can use protein fortified cereals, or high protein vegetables like beans to supplement the protein you get from milk, fish, and meat. Aim for 20 grams of protein per meal, but if you only get in 15 at breakfast, aim for 25 at lunch. You can also increase your daily protein by having a high protein snack like beef jerky. If you are male, larger, or very active you may need more calories than this.

Most people get obese by eating huge portions. A serving is approximately the amount you can hold in the palm of your hand, a fruit the size of your fist, one egg, or eight ounces of non-fat milk or three ounces of lean meat. If you feel you need a more specific meal plan try dividing this intake up over the course of your three meals. Typical portion sizes served in restaurants are WAY too large. You can eat a wider variety of foods if you eat smaller amounts of each one.

Generally most people eat three meals a day spaced apart by five or six hours. For example you might eat at 7 a.m., noon and 6 p.m. If you eat more often than this you will get in more calories than you need unless you decrease the amount you eat at each sitting.

You can find lots of information about serving sizes from reading product labels. If you have not been in the habit of doing this, now would be a good time to start.

How long do I have to follow this diet?

For me, one of the goals of getting banded was to eat more like a normal person. I did not get banded to make dieting more efficient. So the suggestions given above are really meant just for the beginning phases of banding when many people are unsure of what they should be doing. After you get more experienced with your band you will find that you can pretty much eat anything you want, only in small amounts. One of the most helpful tips I can give you is to always eat the protein portion of your meal first.

You will get hungry, eat a little bit, start feeling full and stop eating. It will always be important to make wise food choices and eat healthy food. It always was before. That hasn't changed. It is just that when you are eating so much less if you don't get in enough protein, fiber, vitamins or healthy food during your fewer, smaller eating occasions then you won't get it in at all.

You can still eat junk and snacks of course. But it is likely that doing this will make you feel full and you won't be able to eat the healthy stuff. Personally I have found that eating junk doesn't make me feel very good, doesn't taste as good as healthy food, and can cause problems like heartburn, constipation, and lack of energy. Typically junk food is highly processed, pretty easy to eat, and doesn't stay in the pouch for long. There is no band adjustment (other than being completely restricted) that will prevent you from eating potato chips, cheese puffs, or ice cream. The band is just a tool. You have to make some wise choices about how you are going to use the tool to accomplish your goals. In summary, you "have" to follow the diet until you "want" to. You can start wanting to today.

What do you mean about changing your thinking?

If you have been overweight for many years it is quite possible that you have become caught up in thinking about food way too much of the time. You may obsess not only about what you can and cannot eat, but also about what you will eat. You may think about food all day long. You may be weighing yourself every day or even several times a day and whenever you get a "bad" number on the scale you may be letting it ruin your whole day. You may spend a lot of time feeling guilty about what you just ate. You may resolve to go on a diet every Monday and then feel bad because you haven't actually managed to stick to it through Wednesday.

Making a life long commitment to a healthier lifestyle includes giving up this kind of obsessive thinking. Much of this will occur naturally as the gastric band helps control the hunger that has been driving you to seek food. But there are times when you will have to struggle to give up your habitual ways of thinking about food and eating. You will have to quit using food to deal with emotions. You will have to pass up opportunities to eat when you are not hungry. And you will have to stop weighing yourself every day and giving the scale the power to determine your mood. Rather than feeling guilty about not being able to lose weight you are going to have to learn to congratulate and reward yourself in non-food ways for the positive changes that are taking place. You will have to replace negative self-talk with positive messages.

If you have trouble doing this you will need to seek help from a qualified counselor.

HOW MUCH CAN I EAT?

Your pouch will probably hold only about a half a cup to a cup of food at a time. This is plenty of food for you to eat while you are in the weight loss phase. Since it is important to get in at least 60 grams of protein a day, eat the protein portion of your meal first. If you are full after eating your protein then stop eating. If not, move onto the vegetables. Leave the starch for last. After you are properly restricted, if you try to eat more than a half cup or so of food at any one setting you will most likely have to vomit.

Vomiting should be considered a learning experience. Think about what went wrong: Were you eating the wrong thing, too much, too fast or not chewing enough? You want to learn how much you can eat and stop eating at the first sign of fullness. Pouch packing or stuffing yourself will stretch the pouch, can cause esophageal dilatation and will negate the effects of gastric banding. You do not want to do this.

Frequent vomiting is associated with a higher rate of complications and can cause the band to slip. Almost everyone with a gastric band will vomit a few times. This is to be expected but also to be avoided as much as possible.

Vomiting when you have a band is not like vomiting when you are sick. Usually there is very little nausea. You will have a sense of fullness and a feeling of needing to "unload." Do not ignore these signals or you could end up with your meal in your lap. It is best to stop eating at the very first sign of fullness.

During my first few months as a bandster I learned to spot the restroom the minute I walked into a restaurant, just in case. I tried to sit on the aisle seat when going out with a group.

DO I HAVE TO TAKE VITAMINS?

Vitamin supplements are generally advisable after weight-loss surgery. Ask your surgeon if you should take vitamins and if so what kind. If you have trouble swallowing pills, vitamins are available in liquid form or you can use chewable vitamins.

WHAT IS DUMPING SYNDROME AND DO I HAVE TO WORRY ABOUT THIS?

Some people will have difficulties eating concentrated sweets after gastric bypass surgery. This is usually not a problem after a gastric band. When a person with a bypass eats anything with a significant amount of sugar or fat, they may experience a syndrome called "dumping" when these substances contact the intestines. Common symptoms include feeling light-headed, having palpitations or a rapid pulse, and sweating. The symptoms usually only last a short while but they are very unpleasant so people with this surgery become conditioned against eating sweets.

CAN I EAT MEAT?

The majority of patients will find it difficult, if not impossible, to eat whole chunks of meat like pork or beef and most steaks, although ground beef is generally tolerated if well chewed. It is therefore advisable to abstain from eating meat in the beginning and only introduce this progressively into the diet. Prime grade fatty cuts of beef, goose, duck, liver, kidneys, sausage, bacon, regular luncheon meats and hot dogs are generally too high in fat to be eaten regularly during the weight-loss period.

Other good sources of protein are fish, shellfish and beans. Lean poultry such as chicken and turkey without the skin can also be eaten if cut, chewed or shredded into small pieces. These kinds of food will go through the stomach easier if mixed with a "food lube" such as meat juices, soup, lemon juice, or sauces. Avoid high calorie "food lube" such as gravy, butter, salad dressing, tartar sauce and oils.

Once you are an experienced bandster you will find that you can eat steak and roasts if they are tender and you slice the meat very thin or chop or mince it. You will have to chew well and mix the meat with other textures. For example, two bites of steak and one bite of vegetables is likely to go through better than three bites of steak in a row. However, until you get some experience under your belt these foods are likely to cause vomiting or obstruction and must be approached cautiously if at all.

WHAT'S THE PROBLEM WITH FIBER?

Many people have trouble with high-fiber foods after surgery. Therefore, it is recommended that asparagus be blended into soups, that pineapple be pressed for juice, that rhubarb is well cooked, and that you use only the crowns of broccoli. Dried fruits are not recommended unless they are chopped or well chewed because of the possibility that they may swell and obstruct narrowed openings.

However, fiber is very important for bowel function. You will have to find other ways to meet your needs for about 25 grams of fiber a day. High fiber breakfast cereals either with milk or eaten dry can help, as well as other high fiber foods like beans. You probably won't be able to eat much bread but other whole grain products such as crackers can be a source of fiber.

WHY CAN'T I EAT BREAD?

Some people will have trouble with sticky foods such as coconut, chips, popcorn, rice, pasta, and soft white bread. You will have to experiment with small amounts of these foods and avoid them if they cause problems. If you can remember taking soft white bread, peeling off the crusts and rolling it into a dough ball as a child you will know what happens to this kind of food in your stomach. Anything that has a tendency to form a "dough ball" is likely to cause problems. Switching to bread with more texture or one with seeds and nuts might help. Toasting the bread well will also make it go down easier. Mixing foods like this with other textures, such as taking a tiny piece of bread and then some crunchy vegetables may help it get through the stoma. You can keep up your intake of grains by replacing bread with bread sticks, crackers, Melba toast, rice cakes, peas and beans or cereals.

SHOULD I BE ON A HIGH-PROTEIN DIET?

It is not necessary to follow a special diet after gastric banding. However, it is important to get in sufficient protein to meet your nutritional needs. Generally you need about one gram of protein for every kilogram of body weight. If your ideal weight were 220 pounds you would need to eat 100 grams of protein a day. If your ideal weight is 132 pounds you need to eat about 60 grams of protein a day. This should be divided between your three meals. You body cannot absorb your entire daily allotment of protein at one sitting.

It is fairly easily to get sufficient protein if you eat protein at every meal and always eat the protein portion of your meal first. You will also need to learn to read labels. Good sources of protein are lean meat, fish, shellfish, eggs, beans, cottage cheese, and non-fat milk.

SHOULD I BE ON A LOW-CARBOHYDRATE DIET?

Most experts believe that following a trendy diet is ill advised. However moderately restricting your carbohydrates below the 60% recommended by the US Department of Agriculture and tailoring a meal plan to your individual needs is a safe practice that can have positive results. However, since there are only three kinds of foods (protein, fats and carbohydrates) if you lower your percentage of carbohydrates you will have to increase the percentage of protein or fat in your diet. Diets high in saturated fat may have unfavorable long-term overall effects on health.

The consumption of more protein and less carbohydrate may reduce the appetite, but the type of carbohydrates (see glycemic index) consumed seems more critical to satiety than the percentage of total intake that it comprises. Carbohydrates should never be eliminated from the diet completely. Anyone seriously considering following a strict low carbohydrate diet for a sustained period should consult with a health care provider first. This is especially true if you have a chronic condition such as diabetes or hypertension. Low carbohydrate diets are not recommended for people with certain types of kidney problems.

WHAT IS THE GLYCEMIC INDEX AND DOES IT MATTER?

Glycemic index measures the effects of equal quantities of different carbohydrates on blood glucose (sugar) levels. Many nutritionists balk at the glycemic index because of its lack of standardization and its variability from person to person. However, it is true that not all carbohydrates are created equal.

Non-starchy vegetables and high-fiber whole grain products tend to have a low glycemic index. These are thought of as the "good" carbohydrates. Examples would be green vegetables such as spinach, green beans, lettuce, and broccoli.

Carbohydrates including those found in cookies, cakes, crackers, potatoes, white bread, white pastas, and white rice are high in glycemic load and may result in hunger soon after their rapid digestion. Other examples of high glycemic foods are bananas, carrots, squash, and parsnips.

Carbohydrates that are low in glycemic load seem to increase satiety and contribute to maintaining more consistent blood glucose and insulin levels.

WHY CAN'T I HAVE HIGH CALORIE LIQUIDS?

You should avoid high calorie liquids when you are trying to lose weight. Unfortunately, a number of liquids available to us in our society are very high in calories. These include ice cream, cream, milk, regular soda pop, fruit juices, alcohol, and other sugar water drinks. If a weight-loss surgery patient does not avoid high-calorie liquid, they will not lose as much weight as can be lost if these foods are avoided.

WHAT IS KETOSIS AND HOW IS IT RELATED TO GASTRIC BANDING?

Ketosis is the name for the body state when the body is burning fat for fuel instead of carbohydrates. Ketone bodies are a byproduct of fat metabolism. These byproducts are eliminated as a gas by breathing them off and in the urine. They tend to give the breath a fruity smell. When your close friends and family tell you that you have bad breath during the weight loss phase it may be due to elimination of ketones.

Brushing your teeth or using breath fresheners or mouthwash won't get rid of this smell for long. Taking in some glucose might help for a while. When you stop burning fat for fuel the ketone odor will decrease.

AM I GOING TO HAVE TROUBLE TAKING MY MEDICATIONS?

Most people have no problem taking medicines or pills after surgery. Others may need to break tablets or crush them before they are swallowed. Any well-stocked pharmacy will have a little device called a tablet guillotine that will make splitting pills easy. There are also tablet-crushing devices that you can buy. Some people may choose to or need to switch to liquid forms of medication. However most medications taste nasty so you probably will not want to break, crush or take liquid medication unless it is absolutely necessary. Sometimes you can switch to taking two smaller 50 mg tablets of a medication instead of one larger 100 mg tablet although many times both doses will be almost the same size so that might not work.

A few pills should not be broken or crushed because they are covered with a coating that is designed to keep them intact until they reach the intestines. If you think you might have this kind of medication, you should ask your health care provider or pharmacist before breaking pills, tablets, or capsules.

It is common that medication for conditions such as high blood pressure, diabetes, and asthma will need to be decreased or eliminated as you lose weight. If you have a condition that might be affected by weight loss you will need to work closely with your health care providers to get your medication adjusted after surgery.

Your surgeon may tell you to avoid taking aspirin or other non-steroidal anti-inflammatory pain relievers. That is because these kinds of medications can irritate the stomach and may cause stomach ulcers that could necessitate the removal of your band. This can be a particular problem if these pills get hung up above the stoma or remain in your stomach longer because of delayed gastric emptying. There are enteric-coated forms of these medications. Enteric coating means the pills are covered with a special substance that is designed not to break down until the pill reaches the intestines. As explained above, enteric-coated medications should not be broken or crushed before swallowing them.

CAN I DRINK ALCOHOL AFTER SURGERY?

It is not advisable to consume alcoholic beverages during the weight-loss period. Alcohol is a high-caloric form of sugar (alcohol contains 7 calories per gram). In addition to contributing calories without much nutritional value, you may find alcohol affects you more because you will have less food in your stomach than you did before surgery. When you weigh less you will also find that the effects of alcohol are more pronounced.

After your goal weight is attained, it is possible to drink small quantities of alcohol with your meals.

HOW OFTEN SHOULD I EXPECT VOMITING?

After weight-loss surgery, people occasionally vomit or feel pain after food intake. Generally, this occurs when you eat too much, take too big of bites, eat the wrong thing or eat too fast. Gradually a person learns to take smaller bites, chew thoroughly, eat slowly and avoid certain foods.

Vomiting after gastric banding surgery is not like vomiting when you are sick. It is more a form of "unloading." The food is not mixed with much stomach acid, nor is it partially digested. Usually it comes back up within a few minutes of over eating.

Bulimic behavior is NOT the goal of weight-loss surgery and regular vomiting is not expected or desired. Frequent vomiting is a warning sign that something is wrong. It may be a sign that the amount of fluid in the band needs to be adjusted. Vomiting can also be a sign of problems with the placement of your band or slippage of the band or stomach. Frequent vomiting is associated with an increased risk of complications. If you are experiencing frequent vomiting after adjustable gastric banding surgery and changing your eating habits doesn't remedy the problem you should discuss this with your surgeon. Switching to liquids or all soft foods that go through easily is not the proper solution to this problem. You should be able to eat regular food after gastric banding.

WHAT IF I HAVE TO VOMIT FROM HAVING THE FLU OR SOMETHING?

If you have to throw up from having an illness like the flu then you will throw up. What goes down can come back up. Your band should not be a major problem if you just have a viral illness for a few days. If you have a more prolonged illness and cannot keep down foods or fluids you will need to call your health care provider. Because vomiting may disrupt placement of the band you may need to take anti-nausea medications or suppositories to prevent prolonged vomiting when you are sick.

You might want to consider getting a flu shot if you feel you are susceptible to having the flu and you are worried about this.

AM I GOING TO BE CONSTIPATED AFTER SURGERY?

That depends on what you eat. Many people feel constipated after surgery. This is mainly due to reduced food intake. If you eat less then you will have fewer bowel movements. You will need to be sure you are getting plenty of fiber for good bowel function. Using bran cereal at one of your meals and keeping up your intake of fruits and vegetables can help. Drinking plenty of fluids is also necessary for good bowel function and you may have trouble with constipation if you are not getting enough fluid.

Stool softeners are available over the counter as capsules, tablets, and liquid syrup. Doscusate sodium is a common one. They are meant for short-term use and are generally taken at bedtime with a full glass of water for one to three days. They soften the bowel movements by causing you to eliminate moisture and fat. If you need to take these more than once a week you should discuss this with your health care provider. Changing your diet is the long-term treatment for constipation, not taking daily medication.

If laxatives become necessary, it is advisable to use a liquid laxative such as lactulose, milk of magnesia, or mineral oil. Laxative pills can be quite harsh and fiber laxatives with bulking agents can cause feelings of fullness.

Fiber constipation products and bulking agents tend to swell up when they enter your digestive system. If you try to use one of these products you must be absolutely sure that you take it with plenty of fluid so that the product does not swell in your esophagus or pouch and cause stretching.

It is not a good idea to resort to daily laxatives or enemas because one can become dependent on these. If you are having trouble with constipation that is not relieved with an occasional mild laxative, you will need to discuss this with your health care provider. Remember it is usual to have smaller and fewer bowel movements when you are eating less.

▼

CHAPTER 9

FOLLOW-UP CARE

WHAT KIND OF MEDICAL FOLLOW-UP WILL I NEED AFTER GASTRIC BANDING?

Your surgeon will give you a schedule or plan for medical follow-up. Normally you will need to be seen once a month or every two months for the first year to monitor your progress. It is a good idea to attend a support group with other weight-loss surgery patients at least once a month.

Whenever you have not lost any weight for three weeks and you are making wise food choices and exercising you will want to consider adding a little fluid to your band. If you are losing one to two pounds per week and not having any problems, you are probably fine, but your doctor will want to follow your progress, even if you are not having any problems. It is very rewarding to bariatric surgeons to see how well patients are losing weight after surgery.

Your surgeon may also want to see you yearly thereafter.

WILL I HAVE TO EXERCISE AFTER SURGERY?

Physical activity is important for your general health and well-being and helps in the battle against excess weight. Therefore, while there is no specific activity program that is required after surgery, it would certainly be a good idea to keep up the activity program you are on before surgery or to begin one after surgery. Physical activity will become easier after you have lost some weight and that would be a good time to introduce regular physical activity into your lifestyle if you have not previously been able to be very active. You should check with your health care provider before beginning a new activity program, especially if you have not been very active before.

The most important thing is to be consistently active. It's important to get regular amounts of moderate, self-loving physical activity. Start with a few minutes of walking and slowly extend the time until you can do 20 minutes a day, three to five days a week. Then gradually increase the time. Gradually increase the activities from just walking to walking more briskly, vigorous gardening or working out with weights.

PATTI'S STORY

When a friend suggested I train for a triathlon, I was dubious. At 53 years old, I wasn't in good shape, I had forgotten to exercise for the past 30 years, and I was still technically overweight even though I had the gastric band and had lost much of my excess body weight. Yet, my friend assured me, lots of triathletes are first-timers. I had picked the AARP 50+ Triathlon because I figured if people older than me could do it, so could I. I'd wanted to get healthy and fit for the second half of my life and I knew training for a triathlon would force me to work out. I hated to swim, I hated to bike, and I hated to run. However, a small voice deep inside kept telling me to push past my dislikes and find joy and good in these endeavors. And so my journey began.

Over the next six months I became a workout junkie. I got myself a personal trainer and coach who was with me every step of the way. I told my friends and family what my new goals were. I began to lose weight and feel better about myself. However, there were many days when I would complain that I was too tired, too busy; too anything to do what it takes to train. As the days turned into weeks and then into months, I started to look forward to my new challenges. I learned to find the good in each activity and how it would impact my life in and outside the gym. Swimming felt good, being free in the water, doing quite meditations in my head only hearing the swish of the water. Lifting weights made me feel empowered and I liked knowing that I was helping my body prepare for my middle and late years. I used my walking time as a planning time for the rest of my activities and even biking in the gym was a good experience because I could look out over the sky and mountains and take in the beauty of the desert. Sure, when the coach had practice "mini tri's" I was almost always the last one in my beginner-level training group to finish. But I told myself that on the race day, there would certainly be slower people than me. After all some of the people were 20 years older then I am! Anyway, my goal was just to finish the race and live to tell about it!

I woke up that October morning in a panic, wondering what I was thinking that I could compete in a triathlon. However, my family and friends were helping me get ready and somehow pushed me out the front door. I set everything up in the transition area for my bike ride and run and started to think this was pretty cool being a part of the bigger whole. Then at the swimming pool stating line, I felt nauseated. I had the spectators, the handmade signs of encouragement, and the support of "my" people. I slipped into the pool and heard someone say get going and I stated out slower than usual to pace myself. The next thing I knew I was coming out of the pool and I had finished the swim. That was the good news, although I knew that was my strongest sport. I hurried to my bike and was off in a flash only to soon realize there wasn't a soul in sight because I'd been left far behind the pack. At mile six I was coming up yet another hill, doing all the negative talk in my head that I was taught not to do. I felt depleted of energy and enthusiasm. At that moment I saw my daughter standing on the corner jumping up and down and she ran out into the street to greet me. I opened my mouth to tell her that I just couldn't go on, but no sound came out. She patted my back and yelled, "Oh, Mom, I'm so unbelievably proud of you, keep it up!" So off I went to finish the bike course. As I passed a cross street I saw a man wearing a 'race jacket'. He yelled at me that if I kept my current pace, the finish line would be dismantled before I could cross it. "Take it down if you have to," I snapped, "but I'm not stopping." My irritation sparked a surge of adrenaline in my body. I was determined to finish the race, with or without an official finish line. Somehow, I was coming back into the transition area and left my bike and started the run. From out of somewhere my trainer and now friend, Brenda, appeared and started to walk/run along side of me. She had already finished the triathlon herself and I just couldn't imagine why she would want to go with me. However, she was as hyped about me finishing as I was. She wanted me to prove to myself that I was truly capable of completing the race. She wanted me to experience the feeling of knowing that "I am an Athlete".

With about one mile to go, I noticed the same man who had yelled at me earlier, driving a van. To my horror, he followed me the entire rest of the way to the finish line. As if being last weren't bad enough, now it was being announced to the whole world. All of a sudden, it didn't matter. I was in the home stretch. When I reached the orange cones, Brenda yelled, "run as fast as you can, finish as a true athlete." I saw the finish line and I began to cry. After almost three hours of swimming, biking, walking and running, I took my last step and crossed over to a world I could forever brag about. My family, my friends, my fitness trainers, they were all still there screaming with excitement for me. It was overwhelming!

A few days later, a friend called to talk to me about my triathlon performance. Embarrassed, I asked her to keep the details (i.e., my time) to herself. To my surprise, she told me that a rookie racer who can finish a three-hour race is more impressive than an elite athlete who can finish in an hour. I liked her way of thinking. In the days that followed, I became so proud of my accomplishment. I was tempted to put a "triathlon finisher" bumper sticker on my car. I truly wore my bright yellow race T-shirt with immense pride. After my initial embarrassment, I realized that last place has bragging rights all its own.

As I learned a week later, I wasn't dead last after all. A couple of racers' times were about half an hour longer then mine. Yet my coming in "last" didn't take away from my experience, because I discovered strength and grit that I never imagined I had. I will always be grateful to the people who knew I could do it, before I had realized that reality myself.

WHAT IF I GET PREGNANT?

The period of rapid weight loss is a period of burning more calories than you take in. You will be eating a whole lot less than you are use to. It is not advisable to become pregnant during the weight loss phase. Contrary to popular belief, the nutritional needs of the fetus are not necessarily met before the needs of the mother. The fetus and the mother are actually in competition to both meet their nutritional needs.

Once your weight has stabilized you can consider becoming pregnant, but it is a good idea to discuss this with your health care provider first, if possible.

It is possible to have a successful pregnancy after weight-loss surgery. Discuss it with your health care providers if you plan to become pregnant after weight-loss surgery or if an unplanned pregnancy occurs. You may need to take extra vitamins, minerals, or supplements during pregnancy to ensure good nutrition for you and the baby.

Becoming pregnant may be easier as you lose weight. If you have not been using birth control because you thought you were infertile you should discuss this with your health care providers to see if there is any chance that weight loss might increase your fertility.

If you have a gastric band, your health care provider may want to open the band a bit to ensure you and the baby get good nutrition during pregnancy. The band may need to remain open if you are breast-feeding but can generally be tightened again after delivery and breast-feeding.

WHERE CAN I FIND A SUPPORT GROUP FOR PEOPLE WITH ADJUSTABLE GASTRIC BANDS?

The first person to ask about finding a support group would be your surgeon. Your surgeon may have such a support group of patients who have undergone this procedure or other weight-loss surgery that you can join. The advantage of this is that you will all be following the same instructions. People who participate in a support group are expected to share their experiences, feelings, problems, and solutions. Your surgeon, a nurse or another professional may be the support group leader or there may be an experienced patient who leads the group.

Sometimes patients from several different surgeons will get together and form their own support groups. This is generally helpful but there may be conflicts because different surgeons may vary the post-op instructions a bit. It may also be confusing if patients with different types of weight-loss surgery are in the same group. What you need to know is that there is no one right way to lose weight after weight-loss surgery. There are many ways that work. You should try to follow the instructions given to you by your personal surgeon the best you can. If questions come up during the support group experience then you should ask your surgeon before following somebody else's advice.

E-mail support groups, weight-loss surgery bulletin boards, and chat rooms are available on the Internet. These too can be helpful but once again you will have to be cautious about following your own surgeon's instructions. The purpose of a support group is not to support each other in breaking the rules.

HOW MUCH CAN I EXPECT TO LOSE?

This is a difficult question to answer and each surgeon will give you a different number. The expectations will also vary depending on how heavy you are before surgery, your activity, and how closely you are able to follow the post-op instructions.

The goal is to lose one to two pounds a week after the first adjustment. It is not unreasonable to lose 100 pounds in a year. It is unlikely you will lose much faster than this. And it wouldn't be healthy to lose really quickly.

The research shows that in general within one to three years you can expect to lose about 50% to 75% of your excess weight with weight-loss surgery. How long it takes depends, to some extent, on how much you have to lose. Most people lose 50 to 100 pounds with gastric banding during the first year. Some people lose 100% of their excess weight. How much weight you lose is really up to you. It depends on how serious you are about eating less, getting your band properly adjusted and exercising.

The main goal of weight-loss surgery is to lose enough weight to prevent, improve, or resolve health problems connected with obesity. Be gentle and realistic with yourself. If everyone in your family is round and sturdy it is unlikely you will develop the figure of a supermodel, but you can be happy and healthy.

Remember that healthy, realistic weight loss takes time. Losing a half-pound a week isn't very glamorous but if you do it consistently you will eventually reach your goal.

Is ADJUSTABLE GASTRIC BANDING EFFECTIVE?

Weight loss following surgery is not guaranteed. The amount of weight lost depends largely on how well the patient follows the recommended program. Some people sabotage their surgery by over eating and drinking high calorie milkshakes. They either do not lose weight or are able to regain all the weight they lose.

A Swedish study of 2,000 obese patients treated with drugs compared to 2,000 obese patients treated with surgery showed that surgery was overwhelmingly better than conservative management in improving quality of life, curing type two diabetes, controlling high blood pressure, reducing atheroma (fatty deposits in the arteries), improving rate of employment and reducing costs to the health service. Data from other studies confirm the efficacy of surgery in improving lipid profiles, sleep apnea, joint problems, gastroesophageal reflux, urinary incontinence and asthma

WHAT WEIGHT LOSS CAN ONE EXPECT WITH AN ADJUSTABLE GASTRIC BAND?

Once again, this is difficult to answer because it depends on how well you follow the post-op instructions, how committed you are to developing a new lifestyle, what you eat, how physically active you are, where your band is placed, and how often and how tight it is filled.

Most people are able to lose one to two pounds a week and some lose two to three pounds a week. Men typically lose a little faster than women because they have a higher percentage of lean muscle mass than women, and larger people tend to lose more at first. People who are very active lose more. People who have regular follow-up care, attend support groups, and get adjustments promptly when they need them do better.

Your weight loss will continue like this for 12 to 18 months. Slow steady weight loss is the goal of weight-loss surgery. Trying to lose weight faster than this creates health risks. At that point the body may adjust to your new reduced caloric intake and the rate of weight loss may slow or stop. Because of this "window of opportunity" the best time to make the most use of your band starts from the day of surgery.

Not everybody believes in the "window of opportunity" and some people have continued to lose well into the second and third years after gastric banding, especially those trying to lose large amounts. You cannot tell when your weight loss might stop, however, so it is best not to waste time during the first 18 months by going weeks without loss. If you are not experiencing weight loss you need to change the way you are eating, increase your activity, change your attitude or get your band adjusted.

DO PEOPLE EVER LOSE TOO MUCH WEIGHT WITH GASTRIC BANDING?

I suppose it is possible to lose "too much" weight with the adjustable gastric band but this is very rarely a problem. Generally the body will stop losing weight when you get close to your ideal weight. If you should lose too much weight your band could be opened to the point where you could eat more and gain back to a healthy weight.

WHAT IS THE "WINDOW OF OPPORTUNITY?"

This phrase is used to describe the first year or two after surgery when your body first experiences the reduced caloric intake from weight-loss surgery. During this time period you will be able to lose weight fairly steadily. After a year or two your body will get used to the reduced calorie consumption. Then it may be more difficult to lose.

WILL I NEED A TUMMY TUCK?

That depends on you, your body, your genes, how much weight you lose, and how you feel about how you look. Generally, you should wait until you have been at your goal weight for about a year before you consider reconstructive surgery because skin will continue to shrink for a while after weight loss. With pronounced weight loss, redundant abdominal skin and lax abdominal muscles cause patients to feel unattractive. Correction of the cosmetic problem is an important step in promoting increased self-esteem, as well as providing relief from the various unpleasant symptoms caused by a large apron of loose skin.

The technical term for a tummy-tuck is panniculectomy or abdominoplasty. Abdominoplasty refers to the fact that when a tummy tuck is performed, not only is the excess skin removed, but also the abdominal musculature is tightened snugly. This surgical procedure is of benefit to those who have lost significant amounts of weight or have had several pregnancies and consequently have hanging skin on their abdominal wall or a "pot belly" deformity. By tightening the muscles, the waistline is narrowed. Then the excessive skin is removed, tailoring it to fit the new body contours. If liposuction of the thighs, waist or abdomen is needed that can be done simultaneously. The results of a tummy tuck, properly done, are usually very pleasing to the patient. The abdomen is flat, the excess skin is gone, and the body contours are improved. Contact your surgeon or a plastic surgeon if you think you might want to have a tummy tuck.

WHAT HAPPENS TO THE BAND WHEN I EXPERIENCE PRESSURE CHANGES?

Fluids, such as the fluid inside your gastric band, are not affected much by the changes in pressure you would normally experience when flying in a jet plane. It is unlikely you would notice any effects at all.

CAN YOU GO SCUBA DIVING WITH A GASTRIC BAND?

Scuba diving with a band is possible and is a great form of physical activity. The major air spaces in your body are affected by pressure and descent. A fluid-filled space such as your gastric band will not be affected.

If your lap-band contained a lot of air instead of fluid, your band would appear to loosen as you descended. This is unlikely to cause problems for most people. Ascent would cause an air-filled band to resume its previous size. Since your band should be filled with fluid and not air, this should not apply.

Divers are constantly swallowing air while moving up and down in the water in order to equalize pressures. This air, if not readily belched could remain in your stomach or pouch. Since air moves easily between the upper and lower portions of the stomach this should not be a problem. Your stomach can stretch to many times its normal size. However, you might be uncomfortable from gas bloat if you cannot easily belch. If you experience discomfort during your ascent due to air expansion in your stomach or intestines it would be wise to slow or stop your ascent and allow trapped air to work its way out.

WHAT HAPPENS IF I BECOME SICK?

If you should get a sustained illness that requires you to eat more, your band can be opened or adjusted so that you can increase your intake. Generally a person with an unfilled band can eat close to a normal amount. When you have recovered from your illness and want to restrict your intake or lose weight again the band can be tightened.

In rare instances, lack of adequate nutrition may become such a serious problem in someone who has a chronic debilitating illness that he or she may need to have the gastric band removed. Most of the time it can be removed laparoscopically.

GETTING ON WITH THE REST OF YOUR LIFE

At some point being thinner will be your normal state. You will have reached your weight-loss goal and accepted the new state of affairs. You will know what and how you eat. You will rarely have trouble with your food intake. Being physically active will have become a habit for you. You might even have stopped shopping for new clothes because you finally have enough. People will forget that you were ever fat to begin with and if you try to tell them about it they won't believe you.

At this point all you can do is to enjoy your new body and your new life. Dealing with obesity taught you many lessons that you can use in other endeavors and projects. Please share your experiences with others who need weight-loss surgery.

BOB'S STORY

I have had an ongoing battle with my weight since my junior year of high school. Like many of us classified as morbidly obese, I have tried every diet and weight loss program out there. The problem with all these programs is that they never deal with the core issues of weight gain. They never deal with the emotional issues that have caused you to become morbidly obese.

At one time I considered gastric bypass surgery but I had significant concern about the radical operation. One day I stumbled across the band surgery site. As I began to study the band I became convinced this would be the procedure for me. Life as a morbidly obese person is no life at all. When I was at my highest weight, 385 pounds, I was absolutely miserable. I had to literally roll out of bed. I would be out of breath just putting my shoes and socks on in the morning. The weight on my joints has left me with severe arthritis in my knees. My eating was completely out of control. I could eat a sixteen-inch pizza by myself. I could not look at myself in the mirror. People, particularly kids, would stare at me in the stores and make comments about my weight. I hated to buy clothes because I was always buying bigger sizes. I was at a big-and-tall store getting fitted for a suit in April 2002. I was shocked and dismayed to find the suit that fit me was a size 64. However the real shock was yet to come. The tailor informed me that a size 64 was the largest size his store carried. That was it for me! I scheduled my appointment for surgery.

Mother's Day 2002 was a day I will never forget. We went to a Sunday Brunch with my parents. I could not walk so my dad had brought me a cane my grandmother had used to assist me. I had my band surgery scheduled for May 17th and surgery scheduled on both knees two weeks after that. I did not share my band surgery story with my parents. I sat at our table and I could barely fit in the chair. And I proceeded to eat disgustingly obscene portions of food. I was ready for my band surgery. I was at death's doorstep and I was completely out of control.

The surgery was painless. I felt no pain at any time from the incisions. I dropped from 385 to 305 in two months' time. I postponed my knee surgery because the weight loss relieved my joint pain. My size 64 suit was hanging on me like a tent. I felt better. However something was going on that made me stop losing weight. It has been said the band is the thinking person's weight loss tool. I didn't really know what that term meant at my weight of 305 lbs. (Intellectually I knew what it meant but emotionally I did not know what it meant.) I began to sabotage my weight loss. Instead of concentrating on changing my eating habits, I spent my time and energy figuring out how to circumvent the band. I gained 15 lbs back. In

January 2004 I did some real soul searching. A childhood friend asked me how the weight loss was coming. I told him I wasn't losing and made some excuse that "my body had to catch up to my rapid weight loss." His comment was "That doesn't make sense. You really don't eat anything." Of course I had not shared the news with him of my secret efforts to sabotage my weight loss effort. As I sorted all of this out I made a commitment to myself to change for three months time. I began Part Two of my weight loss journey on February 2, 2004. On that date I surrendered to my band. From that day forward I have been eating sensibly and I listen to my band. The effort I had expended to defeat the band has now been replaced by my mind's resignation to use the band as the tool it is.

Last month I went back to the tailor at the big-and-tall shop for a smaller suit. Once again I was in for a shock. My tailor looked up my account and we reviewed my suit size history. As he was placing my suit in the bag he said, "Oh I have bad news for you. If you lose any more weight you will have to shop another store. You now have our smallest size suit. A size 50." I was all smiles when I left the store that day.

Today as I write this I have lost 34 lbs. since February 2, 2004 and I am one pound shy of the century mark (losing 100 pounds). I have no doubt I will lose another one hundred pounds. I have self-confidence, I have a heightened interest in working toward better health, I have a rewarding sex life, and I have a much-improved self-image. Life is worth living again. I feel so fortunate to be living in a time when this surgery is available as an option for weight loss.

CHAPTER 10

▼

MORE ABOUT OBESITY

WHAT ARE THE CAUSES OF OBESITY?

Obesity is a multifactorial disease. There is no one single cause. Some of the factors that are implicated are:

Genetics and Heredity

The most important cause of obesity is a person's genetics. It is the one thing relative to obesity that a person can do nothing about. If others in your family are obese, then you have a higher risk for obesity.

There is some evidence that chronic dieting and prolonged caloric restriction changes your metabolism in ways that are likely to contribute to the development of obesity.

Currently there is much intensive, complicated research regarding various body chemical causes or contributors to obesity such as chemical messengers produced in the brain and other organs. Genetic research does show that a number of processes don't work as well in obese people as they do in others. These include how fat is burned, the rate at which fat is stored, metabolism, and feelings of hunger and fullness. We will know more about these in the near future as the results of studies now underway become published.

Because genetics play a very important part among the causes of obesity, a person who has genetic obesity should avoid feeling guilty. Obesity is not a character flaw. If you have obesity genes, there is a biological need for obesity. The only way it can be avoided is by choosing a lifestyle that avoids the development of obesity. If you have obesity genes, this is difficult to do because it is contrary to genetically determined biological needs and because we live in a society that provides easy access to high calorie food and inactive lifestyles.

Lifestyle

Another important cause is a person's lifestyle. This includes eating habits and exercise patterns. Americans live in a society that promotes obesity with large-portion, high-calorie fast food readily available. In this culture, sedentary activities such as watching television and using computers at home and at work are extremely popular. We also have wide access to labor-saving services and devices such as drive-through banks and car washes and remote controls and garage door openers. Because US cities tend to be spread out, most Americans drive their cars more and are less likely to bike or walk to work and shopping than people in other countries.

Some individuals have physical problems or disabilities that severely limit or prohibit exercise, strenuous work, and other physical activity. If you cannot burn many calories for these reasons you would have to eat very small amounts in order to avoid becoming overweight or obese.

Psychology

A third cause, although it is not nearly as important as the other two, is a person's psyche. That is their attitude toward food, eating and body weight. We all eat at times other than when we are hungry. Some people eat for comfort, in times of grief or stress, or as an antidote to boredom. Often psychological pressures stimulate increased intake of food. However obese people do not have more psychological problems or more serious psychological problems than people with normal weight. The problems they do have may be a consequence of the societal prejudice and discrimination that they experience, rather than a fundamental cause of obesity.

Research has shown that depression is associated with obesity. However it is not known whether depressed people are more likely to become obese or whether obese people are more likely to be come depressed.

Overeating

However, even when you take genes, lifestyle and psychology into consideration the real cause of obesity is eating too much. You may be cursed with genes that favor obesity, live in a culture that promotes large portions and sedentary habits, and have many stresses in your life but unless you eat more calories than you use you will not become obese.

Metabolic disorders

Very few people are seriously obese because of metabolic disorders or glandular problems. If this is the cause of your weight problem, the underlying condition needs to be treated first. You may still be a candidate for weight-loss surgery even if you have thyroid disease, pituitary problems, or some other metabolic disease that contributes to difficulty controlling your weight.

Researchers believe that in most cases obesity represents a complex relationship between genetic, psychological, physiological, metabolic, socioeconomic, and cultural factors.

WHAT IS THE "THRIFTY GENE" THEORY AND HOW IS IT RELATED TO OBESITY?

People who subscribe to the "thrifty gene" theory believe that the human genes regulating obesity and diabetes conferred a survival advantage in prehistoric man. People with these genes processed their food more effectively and were able to conserve energy in the form of fat so that when the food supply was scarce or unstable, such as during times of famine, they were more likely to survive. The evolutionary pressure of repeated severe famines would favor selection of individuals with this thrifty genotype. The body cannot store proteins or carbohydrates, but only fats; therefore the thrifty gene is a fat-storing gene. In times of famine the fattest and those most efficient at using food survive the longest. The longer one survives the more likely they will reproduce and exist until additional food sources are found or the famine is relieved by changes such as relief from droughts or floods.

In other words, for most of human history it was better to be moderately obese than slim and the potential effects of obesity that occur after you've been fat for years (arteriosclerosis, hypertension, heart disease) were irrelevant because the life expectancy was much shorter. Life expectancy from prehistoric times until 1400 or so was in the range of 20-30 years. For example, Benedictine monks in Canterbury, England in the period 1395-1505 lived, on average, only 22 years from birth, despite having better nutrition, clothing, sanitation, and shelter than the population as a whole.

Another aspect of this theory is that humans have an asymmetric regulation of appetite. There is a strong defense against weight loss but quite a weak one against weight gain.

Obesity is a disease of civilization. The wealthier a society becomes, the more its members eat and the fatter they become. This has been a universal rule for most of human history. In simple terms modern society embodies unrestrained overfeeding and eventually almost everyone will become obese.

In summary, the advantage of having these genes is lost in modern society because food is abundant.

WHAT ARE THE RISKS OF OBESITY?

There are many health conditions and diseases that are associated directly and indirectly with being obese. Some of these are:

Lung and breathing problems

Shortness of breath, sleep apnea and pulmonary dysfunction are associated with obesity. Obesity can impede the muscles that inflate and ventilate the lungs. Obese individuals may have to work hard to get enough air and over time may not be able to take in enough oxygen to meet the needs of all the body's cells. People with sleep apnea actually stop breathing for several seconds, then arouse, gasp and struggle to catch their breath many times during the night. This contributes to daytime sleepiness and never feeling fully rested.

Gallstones, heartburn, liver disease

Obese women 20-30 years old are at six times greater risk of gall bladder disease than their normal weight peers. By age 60 almost one-third of obese women will have developed gall bladder disease.

Hypertension (high blood pressure)

Hypertension is a contributor to strokes and heart disease. Overweight young people (20 to 45) have a six times higher incidence of hypertension than do peers who are normal weight. Older obese folks seem to be at even greater risk.

Heart and coronary artery disease

Severely overweight people are four or more times more likely to die of heart disease than people of normal weight. The main goal of weight reduction for health reasons is to decrease the potential long-term consequences of obesity such as high blood pressure, strokes and heart attacks. Both the degree of obesity and the location of fat deposits contribute to the potential for heart and blood vessel disease. People who carry extra weight in the trunk area (stomach and abdomen) are at higher risk than folks who store fat in hip and thigh deposits.

Strokes

Strokes are also called cerebral infarctions, cerebral vascular disease or a cerebral vascular accident. A stroke is an interruption of the blood supply to any part of the brain, resulting in damaged brain tissue. Strokes have been linked to obesity. Generally the more overweight you are the more likely you are to have a stroke. Twice as many women die from stokes as from breast cancer.

High cholesterol

Elevated cholesterol is often related to obesity and associated with an increased risk of heart disease and strokes.

Diabetes mellitus

Even moderate obesity, especially when the extra fat is carried in the stomach and abdomen (instead of the hips and thighs) increases the risk of type 2 diabetes ten-fold. Diabetes is a disease in which the body does not produce or properly use insulin. Insulin is a hormone that is needed to convert sugar, starches and other food into energy needed for daily life. The cause of diabetes is a mystery, although both genetics and environmental factors such as obesity and lack of exercise appear to play roles. Type 2 diabetes is the most common form of the disease, accounting for 90 to 95 percent of diabetes. Type 2 diabetes is nearing epidemic proportions, due to an increased number of older Americans, and a greater prevalence of obesity and sedentary lifestyles.

Arthritis, back and joint pain

Obese individuals are at increased risk of developing gouty arthritis, a distressingly painful disorder. Excess weight also stresses vulnerable joints, in particular the back and knees, and may lead to the development of osteoarthritis.

Sexual and reproductive problems

Irregular menstrual cycles, other menstrual problems and pregnancy complications, especially toxemia and hypertension are associated with obesity. Hormonal imbalances of various kinds may contribute to, or be the results of obesity. Obesity also affects fertility. Obese women are less likely to become pregnant. When they do become pregnant they are at more risk of problems during pregnancy and childbirth. Obesity in itself is known to lower testosterone levels, cause penile shrinkage and impair energy and self-esteem.

Depression

People with obesity are more likely to be depressed but it is not known if obesity causes depression or if depression causes people to eat more and become obese.

Cancer

Obese men are at elevated risk of developing cancer of the colon, rectum, and prostate. Obese women are at elevated risk of developing cancer of the breast, cervix, uterus and ovaries.

Mortality

Obesity is a serious disease and has been linked to shortened life expectancy. According to C. Everett Koop, former Surgeon General of the United States, obesity is the second leading cause of preventable death in America. People between 20 and 40 years old, with a body mass index (BMI) greater than 35, have 12 times the risk of death of those with a lower BMI.

Obesity related conditions and diseases tend to increase in severity with age. A 20-year old may find that being morbidly obese is tolerable, but by the time this person is 30, 40 or 50 the effects of long-term obesity will have seriously impacted this person's health. A recent study concluded that obesity has roughly the same impact on health as does twenty years of aging.

HOW SERIOUS A HEALTH PROBLEM IS OBESITY?

Researchers recently reported that obesity is associated with higher rates of chronic medical conditions and with worse physical health-related quality of life than are lifetime smoking, problem drinking or poverty. Recently the US Surgeon General announced a yearlong effort to develop a national action plan for reducing the prevalence of overweight and obesity, which is reaching epidemic proportions in the United States. Currently, 64.5% of US adults, age 20 years and older, are overweight and 30.5% are obese. Severe obesity prevalence is now 4.7%, up from 2.9% reported in the 1988–1994 National Health and Nutrition Examination Survey (NHANES) by the Centers for Disease Control and Prevention (CDC). In fact, far more people are now overweight or obese than are, collectively, daily smokers, problem drinkers and those below the federal poverty line.

The Centers for Disease Control estimate that being overweight and physically inactive account for more than 300,000 premature deaths each year in the United States, second only to tobacco-related deaths. Obesity and being overweight are linked to the nation's number one killer—heart disease—as well as diabetes and other chronic conditions.

Americans have not given being overweight the same attention as other risks like smoking, but it is clearly a top health problem and one that is on the rise in all segments of the population.

WHAT OTHER PROBLEMS ARE ASSOCIATED WITH OBESITY?

Obese people face prejudice and discrimination in school and in the work place. Obesity is often seen as a sign of weakness or laziness.

Social opportunities can be severely restricted due to obesity.

Obese people have fewer opportunities for romantic relationships and are disregarded as attractive mates by many people.

Obese people tend to tire easily and may require more breaks and rest than their thinner counterparts.

There are some jobs that overweight people are unable to perform, thus they have reduced job opportunities.

Obese people are unable to fully participate in recreational activities. They are unable to compete effectively in sports and athletics, and they are frequently picked last or not at all for team sports.

Obese people may have trouble maintaining their personal hygiene.

Low self-esteem and body image problems, related at least in part to prejudice and discrimination encountered in school, at work and in social settings are common among obese people.

The disabilities that are experienced by obese people are not acknowledged nor cared for by society as a whole. For example, public facilities that could help heavy people live more comfortably are rare. Many people do not believe that obesity is a disability because they believe that obesity is self-inflicted, although this is a totally irrational belief. Ask yourself, if people had a choice between being normal and being obese how many would choose obesity?

Obese people are often treated as non-persons. The general belief is that obesity is the result of slothful living, poor personal eating habits, poor exercise habits, limited intelligence, or a lack of self-control. Such beliefs have minimal basis in fact.

This prejudicial thinking begins in childhood in our culture. Obese children may be teased at school and have few friends. Some obese children faced with constant teasing have committed suicide rather than return to school.

The unemployment rate among those who are 100 pounds or more overweight approaches 50%. For those who do have jobs, discrimination occurs frequently when there is an opportunity for promotions or increased responsibility in the workplace. Obese persons are often overlooked for those who present a more corporate or professional image.

Insurance carriers discriminate against heavy people. Most health insurance companies exclude treatment for obesity from coverage. Insurers may refuse to provide therapies to treat obesity and will often ignore the scientific literature that shows how surgery can prevent, diminish, and even cure diseases and conditions associated with obesity. Some insurance companies may refuse to sell policies to obese people.

Doctors discriminate against people with obesity. Some doctors tell obese people that all of their medical problems will disappear if they merely learn to "push away from the table." Doctors frequently recommend diet and exercise programs although the evidence shows that these problems are very rarely successful. Would a doctor prescribe a medication with only a 5% success rate?

The severely overweight person faces challenges that a person, at their ideal weight, cannot fathom. Many obese people are on starvation diets while friends and relatives scrutinize their eating habits—convinced that they are sneaking food.

Obese people are stereotyped in books, movies and television shows and frequently made the butt of jokes.

The obese cannot enjoy simple things that most people take for granted—like going to the movies, riding on a roller coaster or traveling on a plane. Even walking upstairs or tying shoes can be problematic.

Because of these problems some obese people are socially isolated. They tend not to go outside the home because of problems with bus, train and plane seats. Telephone and restaurant booths may be too small. Obese people may be left out of social functions that require exercise.

As a person gains weight it become more difficult to move around and inactivity results in increased weight gain. It becomes a vicious cycle.

People with a weight problem often have a negative self-image. They may find it hard to buy attractive or properly fitting clothes.

Obesity is the last socially acceptable form of discrimination in our society. It is completely unacceptable to discriminate against people based on race, religion, sex, sexual persuasion, ethnicity, or disability, but it seems perfectly acceptable to discriminate against people who are overweight. This occurs in the media, the workplace and many social situations.

WHAT ARE THE BENEFITS OF OBESITY?

You may be asking yourself what kind of a crazy question is this. There are no benefits to being obese. But that is not exactly true.

Overeating is fun. If you make a list of all the pleasures in life you may find that the list is not very long and that eating is quite high on your list.

Some people believe that obese people are nicer or that they themselves are nicer when they are fatter.

You may be able to survive better in times of famine or in cold weather or cold water.

People may not expect much of you when you are fat. You might not get asked to do things you don't want to do anyway like help people move or attend social activities.

If you don't wish to be bothered by forming close personal relationships, people are less likely to be attracted to you when you are obese. If you don't enjoy or wish to avoid sexual relations you can use obesity to keep people from approaching you.

You can use eating as a coping mechanism. Rather than having to feel sadness or pain you can ignore and cover up painful feelings by comforting yourself with food.

For most people, change is difficult, even if the change is good. Most people tend to resist change and feel comfortable with the status quo. You might fear venturing out into the unknown. You might fear that some things could get worse instead of better with weight loss. For example, if your siblings are jealous and competitive, becoming thinner might make the competition more intense.

When you think about losing weight permanently you have to think about how you will replace the important roles that overeating may be serving in your life. You may have to find other enjoyable activities for your spare time. You may have to work on your social skills. You may need to wear sweaters or a coat when it gets colder and you might even want to wear shorts or more form-fitting clothes when you are thinner.

People will probably treat you differently when you are thinner. You may have to learn to say "no" when you don't want to do something. You might have to learn to set boundaries with people who approach you for personal relationships that you don't want. If you allow yourself to get close to people you might experience rejection and get your feelings hurt. Of course you could also find rewarding experiences and develop some close personal friends or find a loving partner but you'd be taking a chance.

You might be offered a promotion or a different job and have to work harder if you were thinner. Of course, you could probably turn this down, but that might create other problems.

You may need to see a counselor for help with dealing with stress, depression or anxieties in your life. You might need to work on developing new coping mechanisms. This might not be easy, and it may require a lot of effort on your part. You may feel that you might not be able to do this.

Most people make these adaptations to being thinner quite easily. Your doctor or support group will be there to help you find ways to handle these issues. If you are having doubts about losing weight you should make a pro and con list of both the benefits and the risks of losing weight. Plan ahead for ways to deal with these problems so that if they occur you will have a strategy in mind. And ask for help when you need it. You are not expected to make the weight loss journey alone. Many people find hiring a professional counselor, psychologist or psychiatrist to help them through this stage of the weight loss journey is very worthwhile.

APPENDIX

HOW DO YOU FIGURE YOUR BODY MASS INDEX?

Body mass index (BMI) is a mathematical formula that is highly correlated with body weight. Specifically it is a relationship between your weight and height that describes the mass or bulk of your body. You can find your approximate BMI from a table like the one included in this book or you can calculate it exactly. There are many sites on the Internet where you can enter your height in feet and inches and your weight in pounds and have the calculation performed for you.

The formula is weight in kilograms divided by height in meters squared. To convert your weight to kilograms, divide your weight in pounds by 2.2 kilograms per pound. To convert your height to meters, figure your height in inches and then divide by 39.37 inches per meter.

Body Mass Index Table

Height	Body Mass Index										
(Inches)	25	26	27	28	29	30	31	32	33	34	35
58	119	124	129	134	138	143	148	153	158	162	167
59	124	128	133	138	143	148	153	158	163	168	173
60	128	133	138	143	148	153	158	164	169	174	179
61	132	137	143	148	153	158	164	169	174	180	185
62	136	142	147	153	158	164	169	175	180	186	191
63	141	146	152	158	163	169	175	180	186	192	197
64	145	151	157	163	169	174	180	186	192	198	203
65	150	156	162	168	174	180	186	192	198	204	210
66	155	161	167	173	179	185	192	198	204	210	216
67	159	166	172	178	185	191	198	204	210	217	223
68	164	171	177	184	190	197	203	210	217	223	230
69	169	176	182	189	196	203	209	216	223	230	237
70	174	181	188	195	202	209	216	223	230	236	243
71	179	186	193	200	207	215	222	229	236	243	250
72	184	191	199	206	213	221	228	235	243	250	258
73	189	197	204	212	219	227	234	242	250	257	265
74	194	202	210	218	225	233	241	249	256	264	272
75	200	208	216	224	232	240	248	255	263	271	279
76	205	213	221	230	238	246	254	262	271	279	287

Height	Body Mass Index										
(Inches)	35	36	37	38	39	40	41	42	43	44	45
58	167	172	177	181	186	191	196	201	205	210	215
59	173	178	183	188	193	198	203	208	212	217	222
60	179	184	189	194	199	204	209	215	220	225	230
61	185	190	195	201	206	211	217	222	227	232	238
62	191	196	202	207	213	218	224	229	235	240	246
63	197	203	208	214	220	225	231	237	242	248	254
64	203	209	215	221	227	233	238	244	250	256	262
65	210	216	222	228	234	240	246	252	258	264	270
66	216	223	229	235	241	247	253	260	266	272	278
67	223	229	236	242	248	255	261	268	274	280	287
68	230	236	243	249	256	263	269	276	282	289	295
69	237	243	250	257	264	270	277	284	291	297	304
70	243	250	257	264	271	278	285	292	299	306	313
71	250	258	265	272	279	286	293	301	308	315	322
72	258	265	272	280	287	294	302	309	316	324	331
73	265	272	280	287	295	303	310	318	325	333	340
74	272	280	288	295	303	311	319	326	334	342	350
75	279	287	295	303	311	319	327	335	343	351	359
76	287	295	303	312	320	328	336	344	353	361	369

Height	Body Mass Index										
(Inches)	46	47	48	49	50	51	52	53	54	55	56
58	220	224	229	234	239	244	248	253	258	263	267
59	227	232	237	242	247	252	257	262	267	272	277
60	235	240	245	250	255	261	266	271	276	281	286
61	243	248	254	259	264	269	275	280	285	290	296
62	251	256	262	267	273	278	284	289	295	300	306
63	259	265	270	276	282	287	293	299	304	310	315
64	267	273	279	285	291	296	302	308	314	320	326
65	276	282	288	294	300	306	312	318	324	330	336
66	284	291	297	303	309	315	322	328	334	340	346
67	293	299	306	312	319	325	331	338	344	350	357
68	302	308	315	322	328	335	341	348	354	361	368
69	311	318	324	331	338	345	351	358	365	372	378
70	320	327	334	341	348	355	362	369	376	383	389
71	329	336	343	351	358	365	372	379	386	394	401
72	338	346	353	361	368	375	383	390	397	405	412
73	348	355	363	371	378	386	393	401	408	416	424
74	358	365	373	381	389	396	404	412	420	427	435
75	367	375	383	391	399	407	415	423	431	439	447
76	377	385	394	402	410	418	426	435	443	451	459

BMI EXAMPLES

You don't need to read this unless you want to know the math behind the BMI calculation. If you weighed 200 pounds and were 5'6" tall you would divide 200 pounds by 2.2 kilograms per pound to find out you weighed 90.9 kilograms. Then you would multiple the five feet by 12 inches per foot and add the six inches to find out you were 66 inches tall. Divide 66 inches by 39.37 inches per meter to find out you are 1.68 meters tall. Divide the 90.9 kilograms by 1.68 squared (1.68 times 1.68 = 2.82). 90.9 divided by 2.82 = 32.23 kg/m². Your BMI would be 32!

A mathematically similar way would be to take your weight in pounds and multiply by 0.454. Using the same example, 200 pounds times 0.454

equals 90.8 kilograms. Multiply your height in inches by 0.0254. In this case 66 inches times 0.0254 equals 1.68 meters tall. Divide the 90.8 kilograms by 1.68 squared (1.68 times 1.68 = 2.82). 90.8 divided by 2.82 = 32.20 kg/m^2. Your BMI would be 32! (Don't worry if the numbers aren't exactly the same, this is close enough for our purposes.)

If you weighed 300 pounds and were 5'4" tall you would divide 300 pounds by 2.2 kilograms per pound to find out you weighed 136.36 kilograms. Then you would multiply the five feet by 12 inches per foot and add the four inches to find out you were 64 inches tall. Divide 64 inches by 39.37 inches per meter to find out you are 1.63 meters tall. Divide the 136.36 kilograms by 1.63 squared (1.63 times 1.63 = 2.66). 136.36 divided by 2.66 = 51.26 kg/m^2. Your BMI would be 51!

IS THE BMI CALCULATION ACCURATE?

BMI is a crude measure. However, it gives a quick picture of just how much mass a person is carrying on their body. Although the cut off limits vary, generally a BMI less than 22 is considered underweight, 22 to 25 is considered normal, 25 to 27 is considered overweight and greater than 27 is considered obese. Sometimes morbid obesity is defined as a BMI greater than 30, 35 or 40, rather than being 100 pounds overweight.

There are shortfalls in this methodology. Muscle weighs significantly more than fat and the BMI weight recommendation does not take into account muscle mass or bone density, so anyone who is particularly muscular may appear to be at the top end of the healthy weight bracket, or even overweight. Likewise, those who have a very low proportion of body fat and who are not necessarily muscular may have an otherwise inflated BMI.

Bone density can also affect the accuracy of the result since some individuals have a much higher bone density than others. This is particularly true for people who have been overweight all of their lives, as they tend to have heavier bones than people of normal size who are the same height.

Similarly, the calculation does not consider the different physical make-up of males versus females, the elderly, or juveniles and the BMI should not be used for those aged over 70 or those less than 18. Do you think a 5'9" male and a 5'9" female should weigh the same? Do you think a 20-year-old girl and a 50-year-old woman should weigh the same? Should a steel worker who lifts heavy weights all day weigh the same as a sedentary computer programmer who sits behind a desk all day? There are limitations to this method.

WHY DOES BMI MATTER?

Studies have shown that a BMI of 27 or higher is associated with an increased risk of co-morbid conditions. These conditions include, but are not limited to, coronary heart disease, certain forms of cancer, stroke, hypertension, and diabetes.

Recent statistics show that 33% of adult Americans have a BMI of 27 or higher resulting in over 300,000 lives lost each year due to weight-related illnesses. Organizations like the National Institutes of Health (NIH) that lower the cut-off for normal weight to a BMI of 25 consider 55% of the US population to be overweight or obese. The NIH says that obesity is associated with higher death rates and—after smoking—is the second-leading cause of preventable death in the US today.

WHAT IS IDEAL BODY WEIGHT?

"Ideal" BMI scores range from 19 to 25. Here is another way to figure your "ideal" weight:

For women, give yourself 100 pounds for the first 5 feet of height and add 5 pounds for each inch above 5 feet. For example if you were 5 feet 6 inches tall you should weigh about 130 lbs. (100 lbs. plus 5 X 6). You should subtract 10% for a small frame and add 10% for a large frame. The weight range for a woman 5'6" tall would be 117 to 143 pounds.

For men give yourself 106 pounds for the first 5 feet of height and add 6 pounds for each inch above 5 feet. For example if you were 5 feet 10 inches tall you should weigh about 166 lbs. (106 lbs. plus 10 X 6). You should subtract 10% for a small frame and add 10% for a large frame.

The weight range for a man 5'10" tall would be 149 to 183 pounds.

You need to take into consideration factors mentioned above such as having more or less lean muscle mass and possibly having heavier bones in determining what your personal ideal weight might be.

0-595-66262-5

Printed in the United States
103781LV00002B/8/A